Concise Medical Textbooks

PATHOLOGY

J. R. TIGHE

M.D., B.SC., F.R.C.P.E., M.R.C.P., M.R.C.PATH.
Surgical Pathologist, St Thomas's Hospital and Medical School, London

THIRD EDITION

The Williams & Wilkins Company
Baltimore

First Edition 1964 by J. L. Pinniger

Second Edition 1967 by J. L. Pinniger and J. R. Tighe

Third Edition 1972 by J. R. Tighe

7 & 8 Henrietta Street, London WC2
A division of Crowell Collier & Macmillan Publishers Ltd

ISBN 0 7020 0409 X

Published in the United States by
The Williams & Wilkins Company, Baltimore

Printed in Great Britain by
Cox & Wyman Ltd, London, Fakenham and Reading

Preface to the Third Edition

The purpose of this book is to provide a concise introduction to pathology and to present a compact but readable account of the subject for more senior students especially those preparing for examinations. For this third edition the general format of the book has been preserved but extensive revision has been undertaken and much of the book has been rewritten. Every chapter has had new material added and there are new chapters on allergy, autoimmunity and collagen diseases, gene and chromosome pathology, and the central nervous system. An additional chapter deals with those skin diseases of importance to the student in his pathology course. Other important subjects which have been extensively revised include inflammation, classification of neoplasms, atheroma, viral hepatitis, cirrhosis, glomerulonephritis and endocrine diseases. Every effort has been made to keep the book of such a size that it may be carried in the pocket to provide a ready source of reference.

As in previous editions, illustrations have not been included as they increase the price and size of the book without being a substitute for seeing diseased organs in the post-mortem room, pathology museum, operating theatre and pathology department. To obtain a better understanding of pathology, students should be encouraged to handle and examine diseased organs and not to rely on textbook illustrations.

In this edition, suggestions for further reading are given. It would be quite impracticable, in a book of this size, to give a comprehensive list of original articles. For this reason standard works of reference are given from which details of important articles may be obtained.

J. R. Tighe

November 1971

Suggestions for Further Reading

General Textbooks

Robbins, S. L. (1967) *Pathology*. 3rd edn. Philadelphia, Saunders.

Cappell, D. F. and Anderson, J. R. (1971) *Muir's Textbook of Pathology*. 9th edn. London, Arnold.

Anderson, W. A. D. (1966) *Pathology*. 5th edn. St. Louis, Mosby.

General Pathology

Florey, Lord (1970) *General Pathology*. 4th edn. London, Lloyd-Luke.

Walter, J. B. and Israel, M. S. (1970) *General Pathology*. 3rd edn. London, Churchill.

Systemic Pathology

Wright, G. P. and Symmers, W. St. C. (1966) *Systemic Pathology*. London, Longmans Green.

References for further reading on particular aspects are given at the end of the appropriate chapters.

Contents

CONTENTS

PART ONE

1 Introduction

When a person becomes ill, his symptoms are due to a disturbance of the normal functions of some of the cells that go to make up his body. It is the business of pathology to study these disturbed functions, how they arise, how they progress, and how they affect other cell systems. It also takes account of any factors which make the functions normal again.

In order to understand the mechanisms of these disturbed functions, i.e. pathology, the student must make use of the basic sciences which have accumulated considerable information about normal bodily structures and functions. These include anatomy, histology, cytology, electron microscopy, physiology, biochemistry, biophysics and genetics. The pathological counterparts which have been most extensively studied are morbid anatomy and histopathology, morbid physiology and chemical pathology. A section of morbid physiology which is becoming of increasing importance in hospital practice is haematology, or the study of disorders of the blood cells. A high proportion of the ills which afflict mankind are due to infections with viruses and bacteria, so that a knowledge of medical microbiology is also necessary in order to understand how the microbes affect the bodily functions. In recent years greater attention has been paid to the reaction of the body to rid itself of foreign substances whether these are infectious or chemical. When tissues are damaged, they may develop a different chemical structure to which the body reacts as though the damaged tissue was foreign. These reactions of the body to foreign substances or to its own altered tissues have given rise to the study of immunology.

When a patient dies, the ultimate alteration of function which changes him from a living being to a corpse, is irreversible damage to essential intracellular systems leading to the cessation of his heart beat. This can of course be brought about by a wide range of penultimate disorders, and it is the latter which are usually termed the cause of death, such as carcinoma of the bronchus, or pneumonia, or chronic rheumatic heart disease. The usual way of confirming this cause of death is morbid anatomical, by way of a post-mortem examination, but it is important to realize that post mortems will not always elicit the cause. The autopsy will reveal only the naked eye changes in the tissues and organs at the time of death, in the background of other putrefying (autolytic) changes which are liable to occur after death. On the basis of previous experience, a pathologist may often be able to say that the changes he sees are an adequate explanation of death. For instance, if a pale area in the heart is associated with a closure of the lumen of a coronary artery, he can say death was due to heart failure of a special type (myocardial infarct or coronary thrombosis). However, it is by no means uncommon, and especially in those cases which were diagnostic puzzles in life, for morbid anatomy to give little help in finding out why the patient died. A greater understanding of the events which may lead to the final phase may in some of these instances be better acquired by observations while the patient was still alive or which led directly to his death, as in diabetic coma, surgical shock or electrocution. In some of these circumstances the physician's observations may be the most important contribution to understanding what is going on, but on other occasions laboratory tests carried out in life may provide the vital diagnostic clues.

It will be clear from the foregoing that the best way to understand the pathology of most disease processes will be to take note of a wide variety of observations over the course of the illness, including those at post-mortem if this has been undertaken. Each of these observations will probably represent but part of a frame of the cinematograph of the disease; some will consist at most of a few contiguous frames. A study of the individual frames will help only a little with the understanding of the whole illness, but the more complete it has been possible to make the cinematograph spool, the more complete will be the understanding of the nature of the individual disease process. The ultimate aim of all those interested in pathology is to build up and string together correctly all the constituent frames of the spool of each disease. With some this has been achieved in large measure, with others there are many gaps in knowledge which require clarification. It will be a very long time before our understanding is in any way comprehensive.

2 Inflammation and Infection

Inflammation is the reaction which takes place when a tissue is damaged, provided the damage is not sufficient to devitalize the tissue. It results in cells and fluid accumulating in the tissues and usually protects them from further injury. Tissues may be irritated in different ways, e.g. by infection with bacteria, viruses, protozoa or fungi, by accidental trauma, and by chemical and physical poisons. Bacterial infections are very important clinical causes of inflammation and will therefore be used to illustrate the mechanisms of the process.

Bacteria can settle and multiply on intact body surfaces, without causing inflammation. They are then described as contaminating the surfaces (saprophytes). Some of these contaminating organisms are present on the surfaces of all normal people, for example *Streptococcus viridans* and *Neisseria catarrhalis* in the oral cavity, and *Escherischia coli* in the large bowel. Others will only colonize the surfaces of susceptible people, such as *Staphylococcus aureus* in the nose and perineum, and *Streptococcus pyogenes* in the throat. Organisms may be beneficial to the host (symbiosis), neutral or potentially harmful. Döderlein's bacilli normally colonize the vagina, and by increasing the acidity of the moist surface exert a beneficial effect by making it hard for pathogenic organisms to flourish. The organisms of *Neisseria catarrhalis* confer no known benefit on the buccal cavity. *Staphylococcus aureus* in the nose or *Streptococcus pyogenes* in the throat may serve as sources of infection of damaged surfaces such as operation wounds either in the same or in other individuals (potential pathogens).

Local Defences

It is only when the micro-organisms can gain a foothold in susceptible tissues beneath the covering epithelium and then multiply, that infection takes place. The *integrity of the surface layer* is undoubtedly an important local defence mechanism against infection, but *other factors* exist which help to discourage bacterial growth in the different situations in the body. For example, the epithelium of the skin is always shedding its superficial layers, and sweat increases the acidity of its surface. Tears irrigate the conjunctival surface and contain an antibacterial substance called lysozyme. The respiratory tract is lined in the nasal cavity, trachea and main bronchi by cilia, fine hair processes, which beat particles on their surfaces towards the pharynx, so that they are swallowed. The same tract contains cells which secrete mucus to which foreign particles, including bacteria, stick and which is moved along by ciliary action. The explosive reflex actions of sneezing and coughing help in a violent fashion to disperse organisms away from the susceptible surface epithelium. The high acidity of gastric and vaginal fluids is lethal to many pathogenic organisms and the constant flushing of the urethra with urine tends to wash away organisms lodged there.

If any of these local defence mechanisms are rendered less efficient, the chances of a pathogenic organism to lodge and multiply in a susceptible individual are heightened. An obvious example is the breaking of the continuity of the skin surface by a knife cut. Another way of breaking the barrier is by drinking a large volume of water containing organisms pathogenic for the intestine, such as *Salmonella typhi*. The gastric acid will in this way be diluted and thus become less effectively germicidal.

General Factors in Infection

Once the lining has been breached, other factors, in relation both to the bacterial invaders and to the host tissues, will determine whether or not the organisms will initiate an infection in the underlying tissue. There is a species difference in the response of a tissue to infection, for example, gonococcal infections are non-pathogenic in animals and man does not suffer infection from canine distemper virus. Some strains of organisms will be more toxigenic for the tissues than others, for example *Staphylococcus aureus* is more liable to infect a wound than is *Staphylococcus albus*. Large numbers of organisms deposited in the tissues are more liable to establish an infection than only a few. The portal of entry is also important. If the breach is in the skin, *Streptococcus* or *Staphylococcus aureus* are more likely to give rise to an infection than one of the Salmonella class. In contrast, the latter will more probably establish an intestinal infection than the former organisms. The receptivity of the host's tissue to the organisms is undoubtedly influenced by age and by disturbances of his normal general good health. A well-nourished individual is more resistant to infection than a starved one. This is considered to be an important reason why many diseases such as tuberculosis, prevalent a few decades ago in this country, are not now as commonly contracted. Other states which will lower a person's resistance to infection are a second infection, fatigue, exposure, and metabolic diseases such as diabetes mellitus and drugs such as alcohol or heroin. The standard of nutrition of the infected tissue itself will influence the course of the inflammatory reaction. If for any reason its blood supply is poor, the natural defence mechanisms to be described later will be less able to operate. The presence of foreign material in the infected area will also impede the control of infection. A well-known example of this occurs with tetanus. This serious anaerobic infection is more liable to take root if dirt has been inoculated into the wound alongside *Clostridium tetani* spores. An effect of the dirt is to alter the state of oxygenation of the tissue, which will make the environment more favourable to the multiplication of the infecting organisms.

The Inflammatory Reaction

Infection may be regarded as having become established when the micro-organisms, having breached the protective local barrier, start to multiply in a favourable environment. The essential difference between pathogenic and non-pathogenic organisms is that when the former multiply they will liberate a substance called a toxin, usually of unknown chemical composition, which will irritate some of the host's tissues, whereas the latter, if they multiply, will find the host indifferent to them except that the tissues will treat them in the same way as inert foreign bodies. The toxins of bacteria may only operate if the bacteria themselves are in the tissues (*endotoxins*), or the toxins may be diffusible and cause their harmful effect if they are in the tissues in the absence of the parent bacteria (*exotoxins*). It follows that, while endotoxic infections will always bring about signs of inflammation locally, exotoxic ones could exert their effects on susceptible tissues at a distance from the portal of entry. Typhoid fever is an example of an endotoxic inflammation whereas tetanus and diphtheria are the best-known examples of exotoxic infections. Tetanus exerts its harmful effect on the central nervous system and not the skin (the portal of entry), and diphtheria on the heart and central nervous system and not the respiratory tract (the portal of entry). It must be re-emphasized that the primary inflammatory response of infected tissues to bacterial toxins or irritants differs in no fundamental way from that to other non-infective irritants, such as chemicals and physical agents.

The violence of the tissue's reaction to the toxin will depend on how toxic the material is. If the toxin is very irritating the usual immediate response is *acute inflammation.* If it is less violent but persistent then the tissue reaction is called *chronic inflammation.* Sometimes the rate of accumulation of the toxic product is so great that the acute inflammatory response is overwhelmed and therefore less than is expected. This happens in acute fulminant infections. On other occasions the amount of toxin is so scanty that, although an inflammatory reaction has been excited, it is insufficient to produce any clinical signs.

The Acute Inflammatory Reaction

Much of the understanding of the early stages of inflammation in the skin is due to the work of Sir Thomas Lewis. It is well known that when a tissue is acutely inflamed it becomes red and swollen, it throbs with pain, it feels hot and loses its function. Lewis showed that when skin was irritated, as by stroking it firmly with the corner of a ruler, a dull red area was produced surrounded by a spreading red flare and followed by pallor and swelling (weal) of the initial irritated central zone. This sequence is referred to as the *triple response.* The pathological background of these changes will now be considered.

The Blood Vessels

Following injury there is often a brief constriction of arterioles but this is soon followed by dilatation of venules and capillaries as the result of liberation of histamine or histamine-like substances. The surrounding flare is due in part to an *axon reflex* via the sensory nerves from the damaged site to arterioles resulting in arteriolar dilatation. Histamine and other chemical mediators also contribute to the flare. They are responsible for the weal by causing increased capillary permeability. These chemical mediators may be conveniently divided into three groups, *vasoactive amines* (histamine and 5-hydroxytryptamine), *proteases* (plasmin, kallikrein and globulin permeability factor) and *polypeptides* (leukotaxine, bradykinin and kallidin). Histamine is found stored in the tissues in mast cells. 5-hydroxytryptamine (serotonin) is found in platelets and in argentaffin cells in the gut. It is a powerful pain producer. The proteases probably act by producing vasoactive polypeptides. The protease, globulin permeability factor, a β-globulin, is normally accompanied in plasma by an inhibitory globulin. Leukotaxine is an impure mixture of polypeptides. More recently attention has been concentrated on two polypeptides, bradykinin and kallidin. The former is extremely active and produces vasodilatation, increased capillary permeability, migration of leukocytes and pain. Kallidin is formed from an α_2 globulin found in plasma (kallidinogen) by the action of kallikreins. Kallidin is similar in its action to bradykinin. Wasp sting is an exogenous kinin producing similar effects. Other substances such as *nucleosides* and *nucleotides* formed from tissue breakdown may also be vasoactive in this way.

The flow of blood through the tissues is initially rapid as the proximal part of the capillary bed is exposed to the increased flow through the dilated arterioles, but after an hour or so, it becomes steadily slower until eventually it may cease. The most likely reason for the slowing of the flow of red cells is the increasing viscosity of the blood as a result of the leak of fluid from the blood to the interstitial tissues. The inflamed area is now engorged with blood and thus accounts for the redness of the inflamed area and for some of the swelling.

The Exudate

(i) *The Cells.* Neutrophil polymorphs, the most numerous leucocytes in the blood, normally course round in the blood stream in the central part of the flowing column. In the region of an acute inflammatory focus, the polymorphs marginate more and more along the capillary wall, and can be seen actively to penetrate the wall by amoeboid movement to reach the affected interstitial tissue. The blood monocytes follow in smaller numbers and less constantly. The lymphocytes tend to remain behind. The propelling force for the polymorphs is not completely known but there is good evidence to believe that the stimulus is a chemical one (*chemotaxis*) due in part at least to the presence of antigen-antibody complexes (see page 89) and a serum factor called complement. Not only are the polymorphs of the blood attracted to the inflamed area, but the bone marrow is stimulated to produce more polymorphs. The polymorphs attach themselves to the capillary wall before slipping through because the wall tends to become more sticky when it is damaged. The penetration of the wall by the polymorphs indicates an increased porosity and this concept is supported by the fact that proteins of high molecular weight also get through. Red cells leak out to a varying degree and are usually numerous only in some very acute inflammations which are then termed 'haemorrhagic'. The accumulation of the polymorphs at the site of the inflammation enables *phagocytosis* to take place. This engulfing of foreign material and its subsequent enzymic digestion are the prime functions of this cell. Many polymorphs as well as some of the irritated tissue cells die in the process, and the liberated enzymes tend to liquefy the dead material to form a viscid green fluid called *pus*. The whole process is called *suppuration* and the pus, if in sufficient amount to cause a lump, is termed an *abscess*. If the inflammation is mild and shortlived it will not proceed to abscess formation.

(ii) *The Fluid*. The circulation of fluid between blood capillaries and the extracellular or interstitial tissue spaces depends on a balance between the hydrostatic pressure within the capillaries and the osmotic pressure of the plasma proteins. The hydrostatic pressure at the arteriolar end of the capillaries is a little above the osmotic pressure and that at the venous end a little lower. This gradient of pressure in the normal person allows fluid to leave the capillary blood vessels at the arteriolar end, and for interstitial fluid to come into the vessels at the venous end. Interstitial fluid also leaves the area by way of the lymphatic vessels. When a focus of acute inflammation arises in any tissue, it will soon contain an increased amount of fluid over normal, i.e. it will show *oedema*. This will account for part of the visible swelling of the inflamed site, the increased engorgement of blood vessels being the other major factor. There are two main reasons for this increased amount of fluid in the inflamed tissue. First, the arteriolar dilatation leads to an increased capillary blood pressure, and secondly, through the action of chemical mediators on the vessel wall, there is an increased capillary permeability. The latter will lead to a leak of molecules of relatively high molecular weight, and these will include the plasma proteins. Albumin having the smallest molecular weight of the proteins will exude most easily and fibrinogen least. The accumulation of the plasma proteins in the tissue fluid will now lessen the effect of the osmotic pressure of the blood, and so is an added factor in increasing the amount of interstitial fluid.

The *results* of the increased amount of fluid at the site of inflammation are three-fold. First, the toxin which has precipitated the inflammatory reaction is diluted, which is clearly beneficial in that the toxic action on the tissue cells is reduced. Secondly, the fibrinogen clots to form fibrin, which is thus a barrier against the spread of infection elsewhere. This fibrin barrier varies in amount in different types of infection, so its effectiveness also varies; it is more prominent for example in staphylococcal than in streptococcal infections. Thirdly, certain agents in the blood, which are antagonistic to the toxic substance in the tissue, are brought into closer contact with it. Some of these substances display a non-specific activity against the irritating agents, whereas others may be effective against one type of toxin only.

Examples of non-specific, naturally occurring agents are *properdin* and *lysozyme*. Properdin is a β-globulin which acts with serum complement to produce bacteriolysis. Recent evidence suggests that it may require small quantities of specific antibody to be effective. Lysozyme, which is found only in small concentrations in serum, is a powerful enzyme and may facilitate antibody-complement bacteriolysis. Specific factors produced against foreign substances are termed *antibodies*. A substance which is capable of initiating antibody formation is termed an *antigen*. Substances which do not themselves stimulate antibody production but which react specifically with antibody which is formed when that substance is combined with protein, are referred to as *haptens*. Antibodies will in general only be formed against antigens which have protein in their make-up which is foreign to the host tissues. Bacteria are important examples of such antigens and contrast with inorganic chemical poisons which the body can only counter by means of its diluting mechanism unless the chemical has a hapten linkage to protein. Antibodies which form against the soluble toxins of bacteria are usually termed *antitoxins*.

THE NATURE AND ACTION OF ANTIBODIES

It has long been known that neutrophil polymorphs will not engulf bacteria without the aid of another serum factor, opsonin. The way in which antibodies react against antigens may be demonstrated in different ways. They may clump antigenic particles together (agglutinins), liquefy them (lysins), precipitate the relatively soluble ones (precipitins), neutralize the effects of antigens (e.g. antitoxins) or block the effects of other antibodies without producing any demonstrable effect themselves (incomplete antibodies). The union of antibodies with antigens may be demonstrated only because a non-specific third factor, *complement*, is removed from the serum during the reaction (complement-fixing antibodies). Although in the past antibodies have been classed largely by the nature of their reaction, it is now apparent that a single antibody may produce different actions (e.g. precipitation or agglutination) according to the state of the antigen with which it is reacting. In recent years, by ultracentrifugation and electrophoresis, the chemical nature of antibodies has been clarified. They belong to the globulin fraction of serum proteins and can be divided into five classes of immunoglobulins (IgA, IgD, IgE, IgG and IgM). The first four have a molecular weight of 150 000–200 000 and the last, IgM, is a macroglobulin having a molecular weight of 900 000. Each immunoglobulin molecule consists of two types of polypeptide chains, a *light chain* of molecular weight 20 000 and a *heavy chain* of molecular weight 50 000. The polypeptide chains are joined by disulphide bridges. The immunoglobulins of smaller molecular weight consist of two heavy chains and two light chains. IgM is a pentamer of these smaller molecules. Papain will split the molecule into two fragments containing a heavy chain and the adjacent light chain (Fab fragment = antigen binding fragment) and a third fragment consisting of the remainder of the heavy chains which can be crystallized (Fc fragment). Most of the serum antibodies belong to the class of IgG and seem to be formed as a response particularly to soluble antigens such as bacterial toxins. Only a few antibodies belong to the class IgA, although this is the predominant antibody in the secretion of the

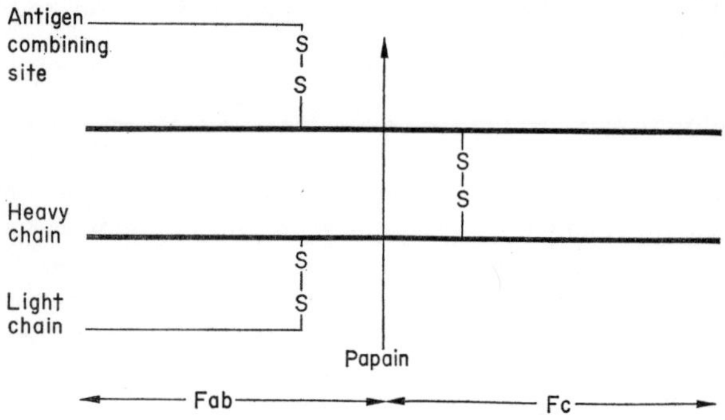

Diagram of structure of IgG molecule.

alimentary tract. IgE antibodies are the so-called *reaginic antibodies* and are involved in hypersensitivity reactions. IgM antibodies appear to be produced as a response to particulate antigens especially when they are present in the blood stream. The serum levels of these antibodies are shown in the following table:

	Normal serum level (mg/100 ml)
IgG	800–1600
IgA	140–420
IgM	50–200
IgD	0·3–40
IgE	0·0001–0·0007

Some of the antibodies are immediately available in acute inflammation, but others take time to appear. In general, specific antibodies take about ten days to be produced in any substantial amount, and so are not available in a person infected for the first time by an organism in the early stages of his illness. He is at that stage dependent on the diluting power of the fluid exudate, and the combination of naturally occurring antibodies and polymorphs. These *primary defences* though more quickly mobilized than the specific antibodies or *secondary defences* are not nearly so effective in combating the antigens and in the days before sulphonamides and antibiotics were available their relative ineffectivity was responsible for the fatal outcome of many acute infections. Once a person has formed antibodies in response to an infection, he is well protected from a second attack of the disease, so long as the antibodies are still present in the blood stream or are immediately produced in a large amount as a result of the second infection (*the secondary response*). The person is then said to have acquired *active immunity* to the disease. The initial response is of low intensity and short lasting. Low levels of IgM antibodies are followed by IgG antibodies. The secondary response gives rise to high levels of IgG antibodies but the IgM antibodies usually remain at their same low level. Infections vary enormously in their ability to produce antibodies which are usefully protective after a first attack. Virus infections give examples of the extremes. A second attack of measles is very rare, a second attack of the common cold frequent. Children in the first six months of life are often more resistant to infections which are associated with life-long immunity than they are later on. This is because they have acquired IgG antibodies *passively* from their mothers who had become infected at some time previously. These are the only immunoglobulins to cross the placental barrier and they disappear within a few months.

Specific antibodies can help to control the progress of an acute infection in another way than by the *natural immunity* process, which has just been outlined, i.e. by *artificial* administration of the antibodies. This was a very important therapeutic procedure for some diseases before sulphonamides and antibiotics were available, having then been often the only way in which the physician could administer medicine to help in treatment. A well-known example was lobar pneumonia in which typed anti-pneumococcal serum was given. Such ancillary treatment is nowadays rare, and the best-known examples are for patients with diphtheria and tetanus, when antitoxins are still given. To be effective, antibodies have to be given early in disease. They are quickly diluted, and if antigen production is allowed to get under way, the antibody levels may soon be insufficient. Artificial immunity of more lasting and effective quality than that obtained by the administration of antibodies can be produced in some diseases by inoculating individuals with organisms or with toxic products. This procedure stimulates the person *actively* to produce their own antibodies to the diseases, without subjecting them to the disadvantages of the infections themselves. The organisms inoculated are modified either through being first killed, or by being alternated so that their inamicable effects are reduced. Toxins which are treated so that the toxic effects are muted are called *toxoids*. In both cases, the inoculated material must be proved to be efficient in stimulating antibody production before use. This immunization procedure is a form of active immunization but is artificially produced as opposed to the natural active immunization of disease. The most commonly used forms of active immunization in practice are for smallpox (living virus) yellow fever (living attenuated virus) poliomyelitis (killed or attenuated virus) tuberculosis (attenuated bacteria) typhoid and paratyphoid fever (killed bacteria) diphtheria and tetanus (toxoids). With smallpox, the virus of cowpox (or vaccinia) is used in immunization. By chance this relatively benign disease produces antibodies which are effective against smallpox.

Summary of Immunization Procedures

Active	Natural:	Infections
	Artificial:	Inoculation with live or dead organisms or toxoids
Passive	Natural:	Maternal antibodies in infants
	Artificial:	Injection of antibodies

Therapeutic Antibacterial Substances

Besides diluting the toxins and bringing antibodies, the fluid exudate in inflammation may also convey therapeutically administered antibacterial substances such as the sulphonamide drugs and the antibiotics. Blood flow will have ceased at the height of acute inflammation, so after the early stages the only way in which therapeutically administered substances can reach the inflammatory focus is by a process of diffusion. This is effective with soluble substances in inverse ratio to molecular weights. Sulphonamides and antibiotics have much lower molecular weights than antibody proteins and the most effective are also very soluble. Antibodies do not diffuse appreciably so it can well be understood how difficult it is for them to achieve their therapeutic effects after the early stages of acute inflammation are over.

Spread of Acute Bacterial Inflammation

The spread of uncontrolled infection is partly due to enzymes within the organism and partly to the nature of the tissue involved. Haemolytic streptococci, for example, spread relatively easily: they have among others two enzymes, hyaluronidase and fibrinolysin. The first liquefies material which participates in the cementing together of mesenchymal tissues, and the second dissolves fibrin. The intact cells of tissues surrounding an infected area form a mechanical barrier of varying efficiency. While most bacteria within phagocytes are dead, occasionally they survive for a while, in which case they may be transported to a distance and start another focus of infection.

Tissue fluid drains away partly in lymphatic channels which empty through a chain of lymph nodes to reach eventually the thoracic duct. When some bacteria, such as *Streptococcus pyogenes*, enter the lymph channels, they are liable to set up an inflammatory reaction in their walls (*acute lymphangitis*) which when in the skin can be seen as thin red lines extending from the primary focus. If organisms enter the lymph nodes and multiply there, the lymph nodes will swell and become painful and in severe cases will suppurate (*acute lymphadenitis*).

Infecting organisms may reach the blood stream either directly from the primary focus or via the thoracic duct by way of the draining lymph. The presence of organisms in the blood is termed *bacteraemia*. Normally the organisms are quickly removed by the process of phagocytosis, but sometimes they increase in numbers in the blood and the patient becomes seriously ill, the disease state being now called *septicaemia*. If circulating micro-organisms settle in the tissues and produce widespread abscesses, a state of *pyaemia* is said to have developed.

Acute infection may reach and involve the serous membranes, i.e. the peritoneum, pleura and pericardium. This is usually a matter of serious import as the whole membrane is liable to be involved quickly and the states of *acute peritonitis, acute pleurisy* and *pericarditis* result. In each case a fluid exudate quickly forms—*ascites, pleural* and *pericardial effusions*. The protein-rich fluid exudate may later become purulent and in the pleura a special name is given for this—

empyema. Otherwise descriptive words are used according to whether the exudate is clear (*serous*) or consists mainly of fibrin (*fibrinous*) or of pus (*purulent*) or any mixture of the three, i.e. sero-fibrinous pericarditis or fibrinopurulent peritonitis. Another membrane which may become involved in acute inflammation is the pia-arachnoid of the meninges, and again it is the rule that the whole membrane will become quickly inflamed (*acute meningitis*). The cerebrospinal fluid will show evidence of this infection in that it will tend to appear purulent and to contain neutrophil polymorphs and the infecting organisms. Finally micro-organisms or their products may uncommonly be disseminated along nerves. Certain examples are the historically interesting though rare virus disease of rabies, and the toxins of tetanus. It is likely that the commoner virus diseases herpes simplex and zoster and poliomyelitis also use this pathway.

Chronic Inflammation and Repair of Tissues

It has already been stated that *chronic inflammation* arises when the toxic agent in a tissue is both milder and more persistant than that which produces acute inflammation. The moment a tissue shows damage from a toxic focus, changes in addition to those of inflammation are set in motion, the purposes of which are to heal or *repair* the damage which has been caused. This means that very often the changes of inflammation and repair are intricately intertwined. With severe acute inflammation, repair features will be minimal; with long standing chronic inflammation they will be maximal. It is best to outline the uncomplicated changes of repair first and then to describe the features of chronic inflammation.

Repair

The body's reparative mechanisms attempt to make damaged tissues normal again but usually a band of fibrous tissue or *scar* will remain at the site concerned, this being the more extensive, the greater the original amount of damage. The scar is least in connective tissue after a clean cut which leaves the edges of the wound opposed and remains uninfected. In these circumstances the wound is often stated by the surgeon to heal by *first intention*.

Healing by First Intention

The wound edges become stuck together by a thin layer of clotted blood released from the cut blood vessels. The acute inflammatory reaction is slight because the tissue damage is minimal. Only a few polymorphs are required to digest and liquefy the few dead or dying cells. Three types of cells appear from the healthy tissue at the edge of the wound. Their purpose is to restore the tissue as nearly as possible to normal. First, free wandering *histiocytes* or *macrophages* move in from the neighbouring blood vessels. These cells probably do not migrate selectively from the vessels. They appear to be in greater numbers because polymorphs wander farther afield leaving the macrophages behind at the site of injury. The macrophages, like the polymorphs, break down the dying tissue, and either digest the products or store them or transport them to the sites of the major concentrations of the reticulo-endothelial tissues, i.e. the lymph nodes, spleen and bone marrow. The red cells of the shed blood get broken down, the haemoglobin is released and split up to the protein fraction globin, which is metabolized again by the body, and to haem. The last named is further split up to an iron-containing fraction, commonly called haemosiderin and to a pigmented iron-free moiety, bilirubin. The former can often be seen as refractile brown granules in the histiocytes at the sites of damaged tissues (*siderocytes*). The yellow bilirubin finds its way eventually through the liver into the bile ducts. The alteration of colour from the red of haemoglobin to the browns and yellows of the break-down products accounts for the colours of the *bruise* or *ecchymosis* which may develop in the damaged area.

If the damaged tissue contains any fat, there will be the state of *fat necrosis*. Macroscopically this shows up as a creamy flecking of the yellow fat. The fat is taken up and digested by the histiocytes so that they will be seen histologically to have a foamy and often abundant cytoplasm.

If, in the damaged area, particulate material is present, which is somewhat resistant to being broken down, the histiocytes often react by producing *foreign-body giant cells* which are large cells with abundant cytoplasm and many nuclei scattered through the cytoplasm. These giant cells will often be seen to contain foreign material in their cytoplasm, a common example in practice being the 'cat-gut' used as suture material in surgical wounds. These cells form by the fusion of a number of histiocytes. These three forms of histiocytes, the siderocytes, the foamy histiocytes and the foreign-body giant cells are performing their scavenging functions in ways which can be identified under the microscope, but there are many histiocytes in repair sites which show no such identity discs and whose precise enzymic activities can only be conjectured though these must include fibrinolysis of the fibrin framework.

The second group of cells which proliferate in repair are those of young budding capillaries. These appear first as solid cords of spindle cells which become canalized and connect with the lumina of the parent vessels. The vessels form a mesh throughout the damaged area, re-establishing the continuity of the vascular systems in the damaged area, and making it for a while appear more congested than the adjacent normal areas. This increased vascularity enhances the scavenging activity of the histiocytes.

The third group of cells which proliferate are *fibroblasts* which appear as somewhat stellate cells with oval nuclei. They migrate throughout the damaged area and are responsible for the formation of the connective tissue fibres which are laid down to form the permanent scaffolding uniting the surrounding viable tissues at the edges of the wound (*fibrosis*). These fibres are very fine to begin with and can only be demonstrated by a silver stain (*argyrophil reticulin fibrils*). Later the fibrils become moulded into parallel bundles called *collagen fibres*.

When fibrous union has been completed there is no longer any need for the increased tissue vascularity, so that many of the capillary vessels disappear. The fibrous tissue gradually contracts with time so the wound edges become ever more firmly knit together. The precise stimuli for all these events are still obscure.

Chronic Inflammation

The vascular reaction and fluid exudate are much less conspicuous in chronic inflammation than they are in acute inflammation. The predominant inflammatory cells are *lymphocytes* and *plasma cells* but in some more acute foci of inflammation *eosinophils* may also be found. Neutrophil polymorphs are few except where islands of acute inflammation or abscesses persist surrounded by chronic inflammatory cells. The process of repair, with fibroblasts and histiocytes, is intimately mixed with that of chronic inflammation.

Lymphocytes were at one time thought to be non-motile and to have a short life. It is now known that they are actively motile and can pass through cells rather than having to squeeze through intercellular spaces. Lymphocytes vary in size. Large lymphocytes may divide to form small lymphocytes or they may transform in the tissues into plasma cells actively concerned with antibody formation. Small lymphocytes make up the majority of lymphoid tissue in the body as well as circulating in the blood. There is evidence to show that they play an important part in immunological reactions particularly in the rejection of foreign tissues as in organ transplantation. It seems likely that they react with antigen and then enlarge and divide to give rise to antibody-producing cells related particularly to that antigen. Under exceptional circumstances they may also transform into phagocytic cells although they do not normally have this property. In summary therefore, the evidence indicates that lymphocytes are concerned with cellular immunity but they may also transform into plasma cells which produce humoral antibody circulating in the blood and tissue fluid.

Healing by Second Intention

It is now appropriate to consider how healing of a wound takes place when there has been considerable tissue damage, such as in a severe, clinically obvious, infection.

It will be assumed that the body defences have just won control over the source of infection. A wall of living tissue will be surrounding a suspension of dead and dying cells undergoing digestion. This may be so great that an abscess forms, and the bulk of the latter may be such that the phagocytic cells are no longer able to carry away the debris. An impasse will then be reached, because wounds cannot heal properly until all foreign material has been removed. If the abscess does not discharge, the body will attempt to wall off the unwanted material by a very thick fibrous wall, and in this way try to live with the disability. A good example of such a chronic abscess cavity is an empyema. It will be appreciated that the longer such foreign material is left in the tissue, the less easy will it be eventually to restore the tissue to its normal constitution. However, many abscesses discharge spontaneously. Since an abscess increases in size in the early stages, it compresses the surrounding devitalized tissues, killing them and *tracking*, i.e. extending beyond its original confines. This tracking will tend to be along lines of the least resistance, and these are for obvious reasons often towards the surfaces of the body. Thus a boil in the skin will point, and eventually so thin the overlying squamous epithelium that it bursts, the pus discharging on to the surface. This discharge can be brought about more quickly by a well-timed surgical incision. The surgeon must not do this too soon before the infection is localized because by inflicting more damage to the tissue he may assist in the spread of the infection. If he leaves it for too long, the fibrous reaction may be so dense that proper healing is difficult to achieve.

When all foreign material is removed from a severe wound, the sides of the wound cavity are too far apart for them to join together by apposition in the presence of a little fibrin as in the case of healing by first intention. Instead, the whole of the raw area transforms itself to a friable tissue consisting of leucocytes, histiocytes, capillaries and fibroblasts bathed in a fluid which may at first be purulent, but later serous. This moist, brown, friable, vascular, velvety, tissue is commonly called *granulation tissue*. It grows steadily out from the bottom of the wound towards the surface being backed up behind by newly formed fibrous tissue, so that eventually the gap is closed by a fibrous scar, as with healing by first intention, except that the scar is usually much more considerable.

Regeneration of the Specialized Tissues

The cells of the specialized tissues have been classified into three groups according to their ease of regeneration. First there are the *labile* cells which continue to multiply during life even under normal physiological conditions. These include the cells of the skin and of the major epithelial lined cavities, and also the lymph nodes and bone marrow. Next there are the *stable* cells which normally cease to multiply in early adult life, but which can regenerate later under the stimulus of injury. Examples are liver, pancreas, thyroid, adrenals, kidney. Lastly there are the *permanent* cells which are incapable of any regeneration after birth. These consist chiefly of nerve cells and voluntary muscle. It is clear that these considerations are important when complete healing of tissues is considered. Wounds commonly involve a breach of the skin. From what has been said it would be expected that skin would show a very great tendency to heal, and this as everyone knows is indeed the case. The epithelium sends tongues of young squames over denuded areas, and these will link up with each other provided the underlying tissue is in a suitable state. We do not know what is the precise controlling factor, but it is known that a bacteriologically clean surface is required. With a large wound which is 'granulating up' to the surface, the gap in the skin or *ulcer* will only be bridged over if there are no infecting organisms in the ulcer floor. If infection persists then the ulcer will persist. Usually the ulcer surface dries when it is clean, forming a scab, and the skin epithelial cells unite under the shelter of this scab. This drying of course will not take place with healing ulcers in surfaces which are usually moist, such as peptic ulcers of stomach. There is a size limit of ulcers, beyond which the adjacent living cells are unable to effect a complete covering. For example, severely burnt skin may require grafting before healing is complete. It is of interest that the sebaceous and sweat glands consist of relatively stable cells and do not regenerate when the ulcerated skin overlying them has healed. The same is true of secretory glands of stomach which do not re-form in the floor of a healed peptic ulcer.

Liver is a good example of stable tissue with considerable powers of regeneration. In certain circumstances, such as severe virus infection, much of the parenchymatous tissue may die. When the infection is under control, the surviving cells may regenerate so effectively that the liver may become larger than it was before the infection. The regeneration takes the form of a number of new nodules of liver tissue, so that the condition is often known as 'multiple nodular hyperplasia' of liver.

The reparative mechanisms in two other specialized tissues, bone and nerve, will now be described briefly.

Bone. The end-result of the repair of an uncomplicated fracture is bone which is indistinguishable from normal, i.e. there will be no scar formation. Bone repair is thus the most efficient possible. When a bone has been fractured and the two broken ends are in alignment the intervening space is first filled with blood clot. This is quickly invaded by fibroblasts extending from the periosteum of the broken ends of the bone, followed by osteoblasts which lay down the protein matrix of bone, called *osteoid*, in which the broken ends become embedded. The dead fragments of bone adjacent to the fracture are resorbed by osteoclasts. The new osteoid becomes calcified but it is more irregular and bulky than normal bone. This woven bone makes up the temporary bony union of the fracture referred to as *callus*. It is gradually remoulded by osteoclastic and osteoblastic activity. The permanent bone is orderly in its structure and is called lamellar bone. The precise mechanism which guides the cells to lay down the appropriate bone architecture is obscure, but the stresses to which the bone is subjected play their part.

Nerve. If a nerve cell dies, the neighbouring cells are not capable of proliferating to replace the loss, which is very much in contrast to what happens in the liver. However, a nerve cell is capable of limited regeneration on the occasion when its prolonged cytoplasmic extension and covering, or nerve, are divided. As the nucleus is unaffected, the cell remains alive, but the distal portion of the cytoplasm or axon of the nerve beyond the cut dies, and clinically loss of nerve function will be detected. The fibrous sheath of the proximal end of the cut nerve will proliferate in an attempt to establish contact with the sheath of the distal end. If this is successful then the proximal part of the axon will flow into the empty distal sheath, and nerve function will return. The axon is not capable of re-establishing continuity of nerve without the guidance of this fibrous sheath.

Chronic Granulomatous Inflammations

Chronic inflammations are said to be *granulomatous* if the cellular exudate includes aggregates of histiocytes with or without multinucleate giant cells. There are several precipitating causes for the formation of such granulomatous inflammations. The most common reason is the presence of a *foreign body* in the tissue, as has already been mentioned. Clinically the most important cause for such a reaction is *tuberculosis* so that, whenever such a lesion is seen histologically, it is usually regarded as being tuberculous unless proved otherwise. The typical tuberculous granuloma or tubercle consists in the beginning of a small cluster of histiocytes with pale opaque cytoplasm and oval open nucleus, looking often so like epithelial or endothelial cells that they have been given the names 'epithelioid' or 'endothelioid' in this situation. A small number of multinucleated giant cells may be present, with nuclei arranged like a horse-shoe at the periphery of the cell, the so-called *Langhans giant cells*. There is usually a cuff of lymphocytes at the periphery of the tubercle. If the tuberculous infection becomes more active, the tubercle enlarges, and the central portion undergoes a characteristic granular eosinophilic necrosis which is commonly called *caseation*. This is because when caseous areas are big enough to be seen macroscopically they have a soft creamy consistency reminiscent of cheese. It is a characteristic of large tuberculous lesions that smaller ones develop at the periphery, the so-called *satellite tubercles*. With increasing length of time the tubercles show an increasing amount of fibrous tissue at the periphery, and if the infection shows signs of being brought under control the cellular reaction diminishes. Calcium may be deposited in the fibrous tissue, so that a healed or quiescent tubercle consists of a relatively acellular, and sometimes calcified nodule of fibrous tissue, which may enclose a core of caseous material.

Leprosy is another disease caused by acid-fast bacilli similar to those causing tuberculosis. The disease is seen in two forms depending on the resistance of the host. A *tuberculoid form* gives rise to granulomata similar to those found in tuberculosis but caseation is usually absent and acid-fast bacilli are very difficult to find. The *lepromatous form* is associated with massive infiltration of the skin and other sites with histiocytes and giant cells laden with lepra bacilli.

The other relatively frequent cause of a chronic granulomatous inflammatory reaction is *sarcoidosis*. This disease has well-defined clinical features, but its aetiology is obscure. It may affect many systems but especially the skin, the uveal tract of the eye, the lymph nodes, the lungs, the salivary glands, the kidney, the liver and the bones. Macroscopically the lesions tend to be firm and pale brown in colour, like flesh—hence its name. Microscopically the lesions are indistinguishable from those of non-caseating tuberculosis. Caseation is a diagnostic feature of the tuberculous granuloma: sarcoid lesions do not caseate, though they may show a fibrinous exudate at their centres. Tubercle bacilli cannot be identified microscopically or bacteriologically and the Mantoux tests in affected patients are usually negative. It is considered that many patients with sarcoidosis are tuberculous, but are reacting in an unusual way to this infection. Brucellosis and fungal infections are other less common causes of granulomatous lesions which may simulate tuberculosis. Crohn's disease of the intestine is another cause which is becoming more frequent.

Syphilis produces a chronic inflammatory cell reaction in affected tissues. Sometimes the picture will be a non-specific one consisting merely of lymphocytes and plasma cells, though this may show the predilection for surrounding the smaller blood vessels which is characteristic of this disease. With long-standing infection there will be both increased formation of fibrous tissue, and a tendency for the affected tissue to become necrotic in a less granular fashion than is the case in tuberculosis. The inflammatory reaction is often still a simple chronic one but at times small multinucleate and mononucleate histiocytes will be present. These necrotic syphilitic lesions are called *gummata* and are nowadays quite rare in contrast to their considerable frequency up to half a century ago.

Rheumatic fever is another disease which produces a chronic inflammatory cell reaction. This is usually a non-specific picture when present in the joints, and in the valves of the heart, but in the myocardium, it assumes a more granulomatous appearance, the so-called 'Aschoff node'. This diagnostic collection of inflammatory cells lies in the connective tissue adjacent to the myocardial fibres. The sequence of the development of the lesion is first the appearance of a change in the collagen whereby it becomes more eosinophilic and amorphous (fibrinoid) followed by an accumulation of lymphocytes and rather hyperchromatic histiocytes, called Anitschkow myocytes or 'caterpillar' cells because of the arrangement of chromatin in the nucleus. There are also multinucleate Aschoff giant cells which have usually no more than four nuclei. The nuclei have well-defined nuclear membranes and distinct nucleoli, which has led to their being designated as 'owl-eye'. In the course of time the inflammatory reaction disappears, and the affected area shows a slight increase of fibrous tissue.

The lesion of the uncommon disease *actinomycosis* caused by *Actinomyces israeli* is usually classed among the granulomas. Histologically, however, it is distinctive in that it is a chronic suppurative inflammation in which may be seen the characteristic clumps of organism. These latter, surrounded by foamy histiocytes, may be big enough to be visible to the naked eye as yellow specks commonly called 'sulphur granules'.

3 Cell Necrosis Degenerations and Infiltrations

Necrosis

For their correct function, cells need proper nourishment, they must respire and they must be sheltered from noxious substances. They are largely dependent for these activities on a series of enzymes, and if for any reason the enzymes cease to function, the cells will die. Some cells are more delicate than others, the degree of sensitivity being roughly proportional to the degree of specialization of the activities of the cell. For example some of the nerve cells survive for less than five minutes after circulation of blood ceases, which is why all procedures to restart the circulation, like cardiac massage, must be carried out immediately if they are to be effective. Fibrous tissue, on the other hand, will survive much longer. Initially, dead tissue will look no different from living counterparts both macroscopically and microscopically. With increasing passage of time characteristic pathological changes will develop in the dead cells which are referred to as those of *necrosis*. In general these consist of swelling of the cell as a result of imbibition of water, and increasing loss of clarity of cell outlines, together with certain nuclear changes. The latter follow one of two patterns. In one the nucleus fades away (*karyolysis*). In the other the nucleus changes from a reticular pattern to one of uniform blackness, and also shrinks in size (*pyknosis*). The nucleus may then fragment and disperse (*karyorrhexis*), or be extruded entire. Karyolytic changes are the ones most frequently seen. The cellular debris is usually then removed by inflammatory cells—sometimes neutrophils and sometimes histiocytes—which accumulate at the site of tissue death, provided always that they can migrate into all the dead tissues. If the amount of dead tissue is extensive then the central part will remain as a structureless, usually pale-coloured, mass. This most often remains of firm consistency (coagulative necrosis), but in some situations, especially the brain, it may liquefy (colliquative necrosis). Necrotic tissue will also soften if it becomes infected.

When a person dies, necrotic changes supervene in the tissues with varying degrees of rapidity, dependent on the state of health of the cells before death, the type of cell, the temperature of the environment, and the degree of activity of putrefying bacteria. The necrosis which is observed in these circumstances is usually termed *autolysis*. Eventually the soft parts will disintegrate completely, the skeleton taking much longer to break up.

Degenerations

Cell function may become impaired for a number of different reasons which do not necessarily lead in the end to death of the cell. On such occasions structural alterations may be seen under the microscope which serve as useful indices of the state of health of the cell. Such changes are commonly called *degenerations* and, in contrast to those of necrosis, are reversible provided the precipitating cause is removed soon enough: otherwise the changes of necrosis will supervene. In other words degenerate cells may either recover or become necrotic depending on the intensity and duration of the degenerating stimulus. The various types of degeneration which can be observed microscopically will now be considered.

1. Cloudy Swelling, Vacuolar Degeneration, Hydropic Degeneration

These are all manifestations to a different degree of the same degenerative process. The mildest change is cloudy swelling and is indistinguishable from the early changes ascribed to autolysis. The affected tissues appear a little paler and more swollen than normal and the edge of the cut surface of affected organs tends to bulge over the capsule. Microscopically, the boundaries of the swollen cell become less distinct and the cytoplasm more opaque and granular. This granularity is due to the swelling of the mitochondria; as a result of their damage the energy required for the 'sodium pump' of the cell fails and sodium is free to enter the cell bringing water with it to maintain cellular tonicity. The changes of vacuolar and hydropic degeneration depend on the amount of water taken into the cell, hydropic degeneration being the more severe of these changes. All three changes may be produced by anoxia, infections or poisons.

2. Fatty Change
(Fatty Degeneration: Fatty Infiltration)

Fat exists in the body mainly in the form of neutral fat in adipose tissue (glycerides of palmitic, stearic and oleic acids) or as lipoproteins in other cells and plasma. These lipoproteins contain protein, phospholipid, cholesterol and its esters and triglycerides. The lipoproteins can be separated by ultracentrifugation into high density α-lipoproteins and low density β-lipoproteins.

In the preparation of paraffin sections, most neutral fat is dissolved and lost from the tissue. Vacuoles remain, but it must not be assumed that all such vacuoles are due to neutral fat, for glycogen and mucin may give a similar appearance. To demonstrate neutral fat in sections, an embedding medium other than wax must be used. The common procedure is to cut sections on a freezing microtome (cryostat) and then to stain the fat.

Visible fat may appear in cells as a degenerative process. In the past, two mechanisms were envisaged for this accumulation of fat. First, an excess of fat may be presented to an otherwise healthy cell which cannot cope with the load (*fatty infiltration*), or second, fat normally present but masked becomes visible as a consequence of degenerative changes in the affected cell (*fatty degeneration*). It is now appreciated that there is an excess of fat in both fatty infiltration and fatty degeneration and that it is all brought to the cell from outside. For this reason, the two forms are not now separated but are grouped together as *fatty change.*

Causes of Fatty Change

The liver has been used to study the mechanism of production of fatty change as this is one of the organs most frequently affected. As the result of breakdown of triglycerides in adipose tissue and the absorption of dietary fat, fatty acids are absorbed by the liver. Further fatty acid is formed in the liver from carbohydrates and amino acids. Most of this fatty acid is esterified in the liver to form triglycerides which are transported to other tissues as low density lipoproteins in plasma. This synthesis of lipoprotein also occurs in the liver. Choline and methionine are necessary for the synthesis of lipoprotein and when these substances are deficient in the diet, as in starvation, the liver is unable to remove triglycerides. Choline and methionine are therefore referred to as *lipotropic substances*. Other toxic agents interfere with the function of that part of the cell concerned with protein synthesis (endoplasmic reticulum) also resulting in failure to form lipoprotein. Carbon tetrachloride falls into this category. However not all fatty change can be explained in this way for triglyceride release from the liver is normal in the alcoholic fatty liver. Alcohol and anoxia may produce these changes by depression of oxidation.

The *macroscopic picture* of diffuse fatty change is one of yellowish pallor and swelling. The liver, for instance, becomes a light yellow brown in colour if diffusely involved, and when incised the cut surface may appear greasy and the edges bulge outwards from the capsule. A common cause of fatty change in the liver is heart failure. The sluggish circulation results in congestion of the centrilobular area and fatty change in the surrounding parenchymal cells due to anoxia. The resulting mottled appearance is referred to as a *nutmeg liver*. The kidney is another organ which may show this change, most likely in a form of glomerulonephritis. Fatty change in the heart is most likely to be seen in the chronic anaemias. The endocardial surface of the ventricular cavity may show considerable mottling, which has been likened to thrush breast or tabby cat striation. This area of the heart is involved first because it is the part most remote from the supply of oxygen.

3. Hyaline Degeneration

This consists of the appearance in haematoxylin and eosin sections of a cluster of eosinophilic spheres in the cytoplasm of the cell. When seen in the proximal convoluted tubules of the kidney it is not strictly a degeneration but a reflection of the increased uptake of protein by the tubular cells following glomerular leak of protein. In degenerate cells, it consists of a protein-phospholipid complex and may proceed to coagulative necrosis. It is seen in the liver cells of alcoholics and in striated muscle in severe infections such as typhoid fever. Here, it picks out particularly the rectus abdominis muscle and is referred to as *Zenker's degeneration*. The changes seen in the walls of some blood vessels and in ageing collagen are often referred to as hyaline degeneration although in the strict sense they are not cellular changes. Vascular hyaline is deposited beneath the endothelium of arterioles in hypertension and in diabetes mellitus. It consists of glycoprotein, fat and fibrin and is probably derived from plasma. Hyalinization of collagen is seen in uterine fibromyomata. The change is due to the deposition of glycoprotein between closely packed collagen fibres.

'Degeneration' of Connective Tissue

Changes may be seen in the intercellular stroma of connective tissues in diseased states. These changes are frequently referred to as 'degenerations', but they must be distinguished from cellular degeneration which may progress to necrosis.

1. Fibrinoid Degeneration

Fibrinoid degeneration is most likely to be seen in collagenous connective tissue or small blood vessels. The tissue stains in a similar way to fibrin, but because the affected tissues do not stain positively with the older standard stains for fibrin, this degeneration was given the name fibrinoid. The more refined histochemical and fluorescent antibody staining techniques now available show that fibrin is in fact present in some of these lesions and γ globulin in others. Electron microscopy reveals fibrillary material deposited between surviving collagen fibres. Fibrinoid change in the renal arterioles is a diagnostic feature of malignant hypertension. Its presence in collagenous fibrous tissue is the common feature shared by the so-called collagen diseases (see p. 92).

2. Mucoid or Mucinous Degeneration

Both epithelial and connective tissues may show an accumulation of mucopolysaccharides which is usually the result of increased cellular activity and not of degeneration. Large quantities of epithelial mucin most frequently occur in malignant disease such as carcinoma of the stomach, large bowel or breast; these tumours were miscalled 'colloid' carcinomas in the past. A common example where connective tissue mucopolysaccharide accumulates is the so-called 'ganglion' which appears in the region of tendons and joints. Mucus may be seen in some connective tissue tumours such as neuro-fibrosarcomata or it may accumulate in excess in the muscle coat of the aorta where it forms the basis for the catastrophic illness of 'dissecting aneurysm'.

3. Elastotic Degeneration

This is a change seen particularly in skin exposed to ultraviolet light and it is found in those patients developing skin cancer due to sunlight. The collagen in the upper dermis swells and becomes more basophilic. It develops the staining characteristics of elastic fibres probably due to the impregnation of the collagen fibres by elastin.

4. Amyloidosis

This is an interesting and still incompletely understood condition. Amyloid is a fibrillary protein which stains salmon pink with Congo red and mahogany brown with iodine. Its chemical composition, while not precisely known, is probably a sulphated glyco-protein. Amyloid may appear without obvious precipitating cause (primary amyloidosis) or it may occur in the course of a group of diseases (secondary amyloidosis). The *primary form* may be scattered widely through the tissues or exist in the form of a single nodule. In this form of amyloidosis the heart, the skin, tongue, alimentary and respiratory tracts, including the gum margins in the mouth, are the most favoured situations. Solitary nodules of amyloid are most frequently seen in the respiratory tract especially the larynx or they may occur in tumours, notably medullary carcinoma of the thyroid. The best-known diseases which may give rise to *secondary amyloidosis* are the chronic inflammations, i.e. rheumatoid arthritis, tuberculosis, bronchiectasis, and osteomyelitis. It tends to involve the liver, spleen, adrenals and kidney most frequently, though it does not necessarily affect these equally and may appear in other sites such as the bowel wall. The secondary amyloid deposits usually appear first just beneath the endothelium of blood vessels, especially the smaller arteries. The first signs in the *liver* may be deposition either in the walls of the hepatic artery branches, or outside the endothelial surface of the sinusoids. As the disease becomes more severe so the sinusoidal deposits increase in bulk, and gradually reduce the amount of viable parenchymatous tissue by compressing it. Macroscopically the severely affected liver will be larger and paler than normal, of more firm consistency, and the cut surface will have a waxy appearance. The *spleen* may become involved in two ways. First the amyloid deposits may appear in and grow around the arterioles of the Malpighian corpuscles, with the result that macroscopically the enlarged spleen will present a cut surface studded with a large number of grey semitranslucent dots (the so-called 'sago' spleen). Secondly the amyloid may form principally in the red pulp in which case the cut surface of the spleen will be uniformly waxy like the liver. The glomerular capillaries are conspicuously involved by amyloid in the *kidney*. The damage to the capillary wall results in massive loss of protein into the urine. The smaller arteries in the interstitial tissue may also become infiltrated by the amyloid substance, and deposits may form in the fibrous framework of the medulla. The amyloid kidney appears somewhat enlarged, pale and waxy macroscopically. On close examination many small pale dots can be identified in the cortex, being the affected glomeruli.

Biopsy of liver, kidney and rectum are effective means of establishing the early diagnosis of amyloid disease. If the precipitating factor can be brought under control, amyloidosis may regress. The incidence of secondary amyloidosis is very much less than it was up to the first quarter of this century because infections are less likely to become chronic nowadays on account of sulphonamide and antibiotic therapy. Amyloid deposits may complicate *multiple myeloma* and are then usually in those sites more favoured by diffuse primary amyloidosis. It seems probable that at least some patients with primary amyloidosis will later develop clinical evidence of multiple myeloma and this should always be considered in patients with this form of the disease.

5. Dystrophic Calcification

When tissue destruction has led to the formation of fibrous tissue as part of the reparative process the latter may at times become impregnated with calcium salts, that is, calcified. Examples of this form of calcification are those occurring when thyroid nodules degenerate, when atheroma forms in arteries, and in the fibrous scars of inactive tuberculous lesions. This form of calcification which is secondary to tissue destruction is associated with normal serum levels of calcium. Calcification also results in tissues when the serum calcium is raised in hyperparathyroidism metastatic (calcification). This calcification, which is associated with bone destruction, results in calcification particularly in the kidneys, lungs, and blood vessels.

Systemic Metabolic Disease

In certain systemic disturbances of fat, protein or carbohydrate metabolism there is accumulation of normal or abnormal products in tissue cells. Many of these produce characteristic cellular appearances.

Carbohydrate Metabolism

Diabetes mellitus is the commonest abnormality of carbohydrate metabolism and is due to a relative or absolute deficiency of insulin. The causes of diabetes mellitus may be (i) pancreatic, following the destruction of the islets of Langerhans, (ii) adrenal, due to overproduction of glucocorticoids which oppose the action of insulin, (iii) pituitary, associated with an overproduction of growth hormone or (iv) insulin antagonists in the plasma. There are two main functions attributed to insulin, the transference of glucose across the cell membrane and the phosphorylation of glucose to the active glucose-6-phosphate. Deficiency of insulin results in hyperglycaemia and glycosuria with alteration in fat and protein metabolism.

The hyperglycaemia is associated with excessive glycogen deposition in hepatic parenchymal cells and renal tubular epithelium. This results in nuclear and cytoplasmic vacuolation. The abnormality of fat metabolism results in hypercholesterolaemia with deposition of cholesterol in blood vessels and skin.

At least seven types of glycogen storage disease are now recognized. Of these, *von Gierke's disease* is the best known. It is due to a congenital deficiency of glucose-6-phosphatase which is necessary in the breakdown of glycogen for the conversion of glucose-6-phosphate to glucose. The resultant excess of glucose-6-phosphate results in further glycogen being formed giving rise to massive accumulations of glycogen in the liver and kidneys. There is gross vacuolation of hepatic parenchymal cells and of the epithelial cells lining the proximal and distal convoluted tubules of the kidney. *McArdle's syndrome* and *Pompe's disease* are two of the other forms of glycogen storage disease in which skeletal and cardiac muscle are infiltrated.

Protein Metabolism

Gout. This results from the deposition of crystals of sodium biurate in the tissues where they set up a chronic inflammatory and foreign-body reaction. The urates result as an end product of purine metabolism from the breakdown of nucleoprotein. The excessive uric acid content of the body may be due to an excessive breakdown of cells as in leukaemia, to a decreased excretion by the kidneys in renal failure or to an inborn error of metabolism inherited as an autosomal dominant with greater penetrance in the male. The deposits are frequent in joints where they cause pain and in the soft tissues where they give rise to chalky tophi.

Lipid Metabolism

Hand-Schüller-Christian Disease. This is a granulomatous condition causing bone defects particularly in the skull where the lesion may produce diabetes insipidus. The deposits contain large numbers of cholesterol-laden macrophages, although the blood cholesterol is normal. The cause of the disease remains unknown but it is closely related to two other diseases, *eosinophilic granuloma*, which usually presents as a solitary granuloma in bone with prominent eosinophilic infiltration, and *Letterer-Siwe disease,* which is a fatal disease associated with proliferation of reticulo-endothelial cells in children. The three are often grouped together and referred to as *histiocytosis X*.

Gaucher's Disease. This is a congenital and familial disease resulting from a defect in the metabolism of kerasin. Large quantities occur in foam cells in the reticulo-endothelial system resulting in enlargement of these organs. Other lipid storage diseases are found in association with abnormalities in the metabolism of sphingomyelin which accumulates in the reticulo-endothelial system (*Niemann-Pick disease*) and a ganglioside (*Tay-Sachs disease*), the latter affecting particularly the nervous system and eye (cherry-red spot on the macula).

4 | Circulatory Disturbances

Haemorrhage

When blood has leaked out from a blood vessel, a haemorrhage is said to have occurred. If the leak is small and is from a capillary, it is called *petechial*. *Purpura* is said to exist if a collection of petechial haemorrhages occurs in the skin or the mucous membranes. If a larger haemorrhage develops in subcutaneous connective tissue, this is called an *ecchymosis* or *bruise*. When the haemorrhage is so substantial that a lump of clotted blood forms, this is termed a *haematoma*.

When there has been a haemorrhage in an organ or tissue, the extravasated blood clots and comes in time to be broken up, the components usually being removed to other situations in the body. The red colour of the shed blood (haemoglobin) becomes transformed to a mixture of yellow and brown (chiefly bilirubin and haemosiderin) before fading, thus bringing about the characteristic colour features of a bruise. When a haemorrhage is very large, or when it occurs in relatively avascular areas like fibrous tissue, it may not be cleared up completely in which case the affected area wlll remain brown to the naked eye and will show under the microscope the presence of many siderocytes in the fibrous tissue with foreign body giant cells, often in relation to diamond-shaped clear spaces. The latter are due to fatty acids from the extravasated serum which are dissolved out of the tissue in the preparation of the section.

Haemorrhages develop (a) because there is a defect in the vessel wall, or (b) because the ability of the blood to seal off breaches in the wall surface has become less effective than normal.

1. Defects of Vessel Wall

(i) The most obvious way in which a vessel wall may become disrupted is by ***trauma***. When a vessel has been cut completely through, the cut ends quickly retract, and, because of the greater amount of elastic tissue and smooth muscle, an artery will contract more strongly than a vein. However, the contraction closing the breach in the arterial wall will be opposed by the blood pressure tending to keep it open, with the result that blood will continue to spurt out unless assistance is given to close the hole. This aid will, in an emergency, be by direct pressure on the cut end, or by use of a tourniquet if a limb vessel is involved, or by suturing the cut end as during an operation. The blood pressure in the veins is much lower than in the arteries so that blood loss from a cut vein can be more easily controlled.

(ii) The vessel wall may rupture because of a ***structural weakness*** in the wall, and this is more likely in an artery than vein. The weakness may be due to a congenital deficiency of the muscle coat (see p. 154), or arise as a result of disease, such as syphilis (see p. 152). The result in both cases is fibrous replacement of the normal muscle and elastic tissue of the wall. In an artery the fibrous tissue stretches because of the pulsatile expansion, so that the vessel becomes dilated at this point; this dilatation is called an ***aneurysm***. When the dilatation affects the whole circumference of an artery it is termed a *fusiform* aneurysm. If only a part of the circumference is involved, then the aneurysm is *saccular*. When a saccular aneurysm is the result of direct infection of the vessel wall, it is termed a *mycotic* aneurysm. The fibrous wall of the aneurysm is liable in the course of time to become so thin that blood will start to leak through the wall, or the vessel will rupture with a sudden outpouring of blood.

(iii) A third way in which a vessel wall may leak blood is through *increased permeability of the endothelial lining*. The leak in these circumstances is more likely to be from capillaries (purpura) than from thicker-walled vessels. The immediate cause of increased permeability of the lining cells is not always clear. Anoxia from any cause is a frequent reason, and bacterial toxins or chemical poisons may bring it about. Dietary lack of vitamin C is a well-known reason which leads to the condition of *scurvy*, but this is not common in this country at the present time because of the relatively high standard of nutrition which exists.

2. Defects in the Blood

Spontaneous haemorrhages are liable to occur if the number of blood platelets falls to a low level (thrombocytopenia) or if an abnormality develops in the coagulation mechanism, as for example in haemophilia. Thrombocytopenia leads to purpura, which shows that the integrity of the capillary endothelium must be partly dependent on the number of circulating platelets. The platelets exert their haemostatic effect in two ways. They clump together and seal off breaches that may develop in the capillary wall, and they have a vasoconstrictive action as a result of the 5-hydroxytryptamine (serotonin) which is present on their surface.

Defects in the blood coagulation mechanism do not usually lead to purpura but to a diffuse and persistent oozing of blood. This may develop spontaneously or become evident as a result of a traumatic episode such as dental extraction which would be quickly followed by normal haemostasis in a normal person.

Another cause of bleeding is abnormal fibrinolysis. Normally there exists a system whereby small amounts of fibrin are destroyed by the proteolytic enzyme *plasmin.* In certain disease states the fibrinolytic system becomes abnormally activated so that it not only destroys fibrin as it forms in clots but it also destroys fibrinogen, resulting in a coagulation defect

Thrombosis

The endothelial lining of the blood vessels consists normally of a smooth surface which enables the blood within to circulate without appreciable coagulation taking place. Once the endothelial lining becomes roughened, as for example following trauma, a chain of events takes place in the blood which leads to the formation of a solid mass of tissue at the roughened area, the primary purpose of which is to repair the breach in the endothelium. This mass which is formed from the elements in the blood is termed a *thrombus.* The first thing to happen at the damaged endothelial surface is the formation of a mass of clumped platelets. These elements will always adhere to roughened surfaces and, when adherent, will alter in texture so that they become more sticky and more amorphous. This platelet clump is of pale colour to the naked eye and is commonly termed a *white thrombus*. This appears to be all that is necessary to seal off small wounds of vascular endothelium, the platelets' surface being quickly covered by endothelial cells budded off from the surrounding intact endothelium. This endothelial spread is very rapid in normal circumstances. If the damaged area is extensive, the white thrombus will continue to grow into the lumen of the vessel in a spiral fashion. This will create eddies in the flowing blood, which enables the concentration of blood thromboplastin to build up to a sufficiently high level to initiate the precipitation of fibrin on to the surface of the platelets. The fibrin network enmeshes red cells among the fibres and provides a roughened surface for more platelet deposition, with the result that the thrombus may become so big as to occlude the lumen of the vessel. This *red thrombus*, when seen macroscopically, will look a dull chocolate brown with paler brown ribbing—the lines of Zahn—and can be fairly easily broken up. Under the microscope, the characteristic picture is one of alternate layers of hyaline pale pink platelet thrombus and of darker pink fibrin fibrils surrounding red cells. The white cells chiefly palisade the platelet layers, but may also be scattered through the fibrin network.

Factors Influencing Thrombus Formation

Important factors which favour the production of red thrombi are damaged endothelium, slowing of the circulation, and increased coagulability of the blood.

(i) *Damaged Endothelium*

The significance of this has already been discussed. The changes in the endothelium may be traumatic as in crush injuries or from suture material in vascular surgery, or the damage may result from the injection of irritating chemicals. Anoxia is also an important factor in veins. In arteries atheroma and mechanical stresses are the commonest causes of endothelial damage.

(ii) *Slowing of the Circulation*

Whenever platelet thrombi start to form, the normal coagulation process is always initiated, but if the flow of blood is fast, the blood thromboplastin which is formed is swept away and diluted in the process. In addition, these small amounts will be neutralized by the natural anticoagulant substances which circulate in the blood. It is for this reason that red thrombi only develop slowly, if at all, in arteries. In veins, by contrast, the flow is normally slower and becomes even slower still under certain clinical conditions, such as congestive cardiac failure, or locally in varicose veins. The flow of blood in the deep veins of the leg is largely dependent on the pumping action of the leg muscles during exercise. The inactivity associated with lying in bed will thus slow the vein flow in the legs and this is especially true if the patient is so ill that he does not move around much. Thus it is not surprising that red thrombi are much commoner and more extensive in veins than arteries and that the deep leg veins are chiefly affected especially in ill patients in bed. The slowing of the blood flow initiates a vicious circle of tendency to thrombus formation, because it damages the endothelial lining cells by making them more anoxic.

Increased viscosity of blood will also tend to reduce blood flow. This can arise either when red cells are increased relative to the plasma (polycythaemia) or when the plasma volume decreases relative to red cells (dehydration).

(iii) *Increased Coagulability of the Blood*

There is evidence that blood coagulation proceeds more quickly after operations. There is an immediate increase in numbers of platelets which may be two- or three-fold. These platelets become more sticky than normal, and an increase in activity of other clotting factors has been demonstrated. Blood also tends to coagulate more easily than normal in some blood diseases, of which the most prone is polycythaemia in which platelets are often increased in numbers. The fact that the blood is more viscous, as has just been mentioned, is contributory in this disease.

Sequels of Thrombosis

(i) *Resolution*

Not all thrombi persist for any length of time. Platelet clumps forming a white thrombus may be broken up by phosphatases released from the vessel wall. When fibrin strands form, they may be digested by the fibrinolytic activity of either the plasma or leukocytes. Contraction of the thrombus will lead to it shrinking back to occupy only part of the lumen of the vessel.

(ii) *Organization*

If the thrombus is not dissolved then organization will occur. By this means continuity of the vascular lumen may be restored. Capillaries, fibroblasts and histiocytes move in from the intima of the vessel in order to digest and remove the components of the blood which form the thrombus and to replace it with varying amounts of fibrous stroma. The endothelial cells spread over and cover the organizing thrombus on its luminal side. Thus the thrombus which only partially occludes the lumen ends up as a fibrous plaque in the wall of the vessel covered by endothelium. The thrombus which occludes the lumen completely becomes penetrated by capillaries growing in from the vessel wall. These gradually dilate so that they establish continuity at a number of points and the organized occlusive thrombus tends more often than not to have a number of small channels rather than a single one. It follows that this reconstructed blood vessel will be less efficient than normal.

(iii) *Effects on the Part Supplied by the Blood Vessel*

The effect of thrombus formation on the part supplied by a vessel will depend on whether this is the only vessel of supply to the part or whether it anastomoses with other channels which can take over its function if it is blocked. Individual arteries may, in certain situations, be the only vessels of supply—the so-called *end-arteries*, but veins are virtually never end-veins. Examples of end-arteries are seen in the brain, heart, spleen, kidney and retina.

Another factor which will determine the effect on the part is the speed of the narrowing of the lumen by the thrombus. If a thrombus forms rapidly in an end-artery the blood supply is suddenly cut off from the part supplied and its component cells will die. Necrosis of tissue ensuing under such conditions is referred to as an *infarct*. If a thrombus forms more slowly in an artery or only partly occludes the vessel lumen, then the reduction of blood supply to the tissue supplied will take place slowly and may never be complete. This will lead to death or atrophy of a few cells at a time, and to *replacement fibrosis*. The fibrosis is often more limited than might be expected because the neighbouring unaffected vessels have had time to form anastomotic channels and thus to take over some of the blood supply to the part.

When a vein is rapidly occluded by a thrombus the effect on the part supplied will depend on the adequacy of the collateral circulation which is, in most instances, good. In these circumstances the most that will take place will be a transient congestion and oedema of the part. On those occasions when the collateral circulation is inadequate, the affected tissue becomes engorged with blood and will subsequently die for lack of proper nutrition (venous infarction).

(iv) *Embolism*

Thrombi are friable unless they are undergoing organization, so that fragments or *emboli* are liable to break off into the blood stream. Arterial emboli are rarely large, but if they lodge in those organs supplied by end-arteries such as the spleen, kidney, heart and brain, they will lead to the formation of infarcts. Venous emboli can be very large. When a small vein, such as one of the intramuscular branches in the leg, becomes occluded by thrombus the blood becomes stationary in the vessel on either side of the block and so will coagulate. That in the distal portion will eventually organize, but the clot attached to the thrombus in the proximal part of the vein often extends to the junction with another vessel leading into a larger vein. The free end of the 'propagated thrombus' will be buffeted by the blood flowing freely by in the adjacent patent vein, and is liable to be broken off, to be transported through the right side of the heart into the pulmonary artery system. Here they may block the major branches of the pulmonary artery and cause sudden death, or they may block more peripheral branches. The effects will then depend on the adequacy of the collateral circulation in this area. If this is impaired, pulmonary infarction will ensue.

Embolism

An embolus is a particulate mass circulating in a vascular channel, and is not a normal component of the circulating fluid. We have seen in the previous section that a detached fragment of thrombus from a vessel wall is a cause of embolism in blood vessels. Emboli from thrombosed veins, reaching the pulmonary artery tree, assume great importance in clinical medicine because of the fatal outcome associated with the larger ones. The veins most frequently involved are the deep veins of the legs, the others next most affected are the veins draining the pelvic organs. The deep veins of the legs are liable to thrombose when the muscles are inactive, and this situation is most likely to arise, as has already been stated, when a patient lies in bed for any length of time. The pelvic veins become thrombosed after operations on pelvic organs, when trauma and infection may be important initiating factors. The most common arterial emboli are detached fragments of atheromatous plaques. Those which break away from plaques in the carotid arteries are now considered to be the common cause of recurrent cerebral infarction.

Emboli arise from other sources as well as from thrombi in vessel walls; examples follow. (1) Vegetations on the heart valves or adjacent endothelial surfaces. The ones most likely to fragment are the vegetations of either subacute or acute bacterial endocarditis. The former differ from the latter in that the infarcts which follow embolization are not liable to become septic. (2) Thrombi on the endocardial surfaces of the ventricles, particularly the left ventricle. The most common cause of these is an underlying myocardial infarct. (3) Thrombi in the auricular appendages. These are prone to develop in the fibrillating heart, as in chronic rheumatic heart disease and thyrotoxicosis. (4) Neoplastic emboli. Fragments of malignant tumour are liable to infiltrate venous and lymphatic channels and then break off to lodge elsewhere in the body. This mechanism is of great importance in the spread of malignant tumours. (5) Fat emboli. These are most likely to occur after a fracture of bone. Fat from the fatty marrow finds its way into the ruptured venous sinuses and gets transported to the pulmonary capillaries and through them to other tissues in the body such as the brain. (6) Air emboli. Air may be transported along veins to the heart. This can happen after superficial wounds to the veins of the neck, when the negative pressure produced by breathing sucks the air in. It is also a complication of faulty transfusion technique. A large quantity of air has to be sucked in before ill effects are observed, and these arise as a result of frothing of blood in the right ventricle leading to obstruction of blood flow into the lungs. Caisson disease is closely related to air embolism. Inert gases, such as nitrogen, dissolve in the blood under the high pressure of air breathed by divers. If the pressure is rapidly reduced, this nitrogen bubbles out of solution giving gas emboli and the clinical effects of 'the bends' (7). Amniotic embolism may occur during labour and gives rise to respiratory distress or coagulation abnormalities including defibrination due to the thromboplastic activity of the amniotic fluid. (8) Parasite emboli may block small vessels such as the cerebral vessels in malaria (p. 63).

Results of Embolism

Some of the effects have already been mentioned in the section on thrombosis. Emboli arising from the left auricle or ventricle, or from the mitral or aortic valves, or from the arterial lumina, will be propagated further into the arterial tree until they impact. Whether clinical effects will arise from such impaction will depend on the size of the particle and the state of the collateral circulation. If effects do become evident, these are most likely to be due to infarction of the organ involved. Sites where symptoms are liable to become manifest are the brain (e.g. hemiplegia), the kidney (haematuria) and the spleen (splenic pain). A large detached thrombus becoming wedged across the bifurcation of the aorta is called a 'saddle' embolus. This is usually of intracardiac origin and requires urgent surgical removal if the legs are to be saved.

Emboli arising in the veins are propagated to the lungs or liver. As thrombi are most likely in leg or pelvic veins, the lungs are the organs most likely to receive thrombotic emboli. The effects in the lungs will depend on the size of the emboli, and the circulatory state of the lungs. The largest emboli will impact in the main pulmonary arteries and will cause death within a few seconds as a result of the sudden cut-off of blood supply to the lungs and beyond. The smallest emboli may produce no symptoms. Intermediate ones will produce pulmonary infarcts, and the size of these will depend on whether there is pulmonary venous congestion or not. The more congested the lung the larger will the infarct be following occlusion in any one situation in the pulmonary artery tree. When lungs are not congested, the blood supply through the bronchial artery system may be sufficient to maintain the proper nutrition of the lung involved by the embolus.

If thrombotic emboli are infected particles, abscesses are liable to develop at the site of impaction (pyaemic abscesses). This occurs in septic thrombophlebitis, in portal pyaemia, and in acute bacterial endocarditis. When malignant cells embolize, they may either die or continue to grow where impacted, and form masses of secondary growth or *metastases*. The conditions which favour the continued growth of neoplastic emboli are little understood. Only a small proportion of disseminated malignant cells become metastases, and the latter are more common in certain organs than others.

Ischaemia

The tissues of the body are completely dependent on an adequate supply of oxygenated blood for their proper nutrition. Whenever this supply becomes inadequate, the tissue is said to become *ischaemic*. The more active tissues suffer earlier from lack of oxygen (anoxia) than the less active. For example, epithelial cells are more susceptible than the connective tissues, and the neurones of the brain are the most susceptible of all cells, some of which will show evidence of functional disturbances after only a few seconds of oxygen deprivation. It is clear therefore, that the effect of ischaemia on the tissues of the body will depend on (a) the extent of tissue exposed to anoxia, (b) the susceptibility of the part to anoxia, (c) the severity of the anoxia, and (d) the duration of the anoxia.

The anoxia may be general or local. *General anoxia* is brought about when there is inadequate gaseous exchange in the lungs, such as in cardiovascular and respiratory disease, or if cellular respiration is interfered with, such as in cyanide poisoning, or if red cells can no longer effectively transport oxygen, such as in anaemia and carbon monoxide poisoning. The results of *local anoxia* if sustained for sufficiently long are (a) replacement fibrosis and (b) infarction.

1. Replacement Fibrosis

Replacement fibrosis comes about in organs submitted to persistent mild anoxia. As has already been stated, an important site for this change is in the heart. If the blood supply in the heart becomes reduced slowly as a result of atheromatous disease in the coronary arteries, the myocardial fibres will die in the affected area and be replaced by fibrous tissue which can still survive under the anoxic conditions. Similar changes can occur in the kidney (ischaemic atrophy), liver (cirrhosis) and in the brain (replacement gliosis).

2. Infarction

An infarct is a sharply defined, often wedge-shaped, area of necrosis resulting from acute and complete anoxia following obstruction to the local circulation. It has already been pointed out that this obstruction occurs when either an atheromatous artery becomes completely thrombosed, or an artery becomes impacted with an embolus, and these are the common causes of infarction. The obstruction can be brought about in other ways. For example, torsion or twisting of a pedicle containing the blood supply may occur in a loop of intestine (volvulus), in an ovarian cyst, or in a testicle. The infarction in these circumstances is usually haemorrhagic, because the veins become more easily obstructed than the arteries. Accidental infarction may be brought about by ligature of an artery at operation.

When a vessel lumen is obstructed, the extent of infarction of the tissue involved will depend on the blood supply to the area. As has already been mentioned, if sufficient collateral blood channels exist, the tissue is much less likely to become necrotic than otherwise. The liver and lungs are two organs which receive a double blood supply so that if these organs are otherwise normal, occlusion of a branch of one of the vessels may produce no change. However, infarcts become a common complication in the lung if the circulatory system is abnormal, as in congestive cardiac failure. In the heart, kidney, spleen and brain, collateral circulations are not normally so well developed, so that infarcts more easily develop. In the case of the heart, the slowly progressive narrowing which occurs in the atheromatous arteries tends to open up channels of communication between neighbouring branches, so that infarcts are often smaller than expected following the occlusion of an atheromatous artery.

The changes of infarction are exemplified by those occurring in myocardial infarction. Within the first 12 hours little change is to be seen which explains why the muscle appears normal at autopsy in cases of sudden death due to myocardial infarction. However changes are detectable by histochemistry and by electron microscopy within a few hours. By 24 hours there is leakage of blood by backflow from vessels into the infarct. The tissue becomes pale due to accumulation of fluid between muscle fibres. Over the next 2 to 4 days the infarcted area becomes more clearly demarcated. It is yellow due to the breakdown of blood pigments which are ingested by infiltrating polymorphs and histiocytes. The infarct is soft because of the enzymic action of these infiltrating cells and interstitial oedema. There is a surrounding hyperaemic zone. By 10 days the infarct is very soft (*myomalacia cordis*) and the yellow discoloration is most noticeable. Rupture of the infarct is now common. Over the following 6 weeks, in those who survive, there is progressive fibrosis from the margins inwards. The dead muscle is replaced by firm, grey scar tissue which is thinner than the original muscle.

In those sites where the tissue is of loose texture as in the lung and intestine, the leakage of blood into the tissues causes them to become dark and stuffed with blood. There is no compression of damaged vessels as in solid organs, so the pallor is not seen until the infarct has organized and been replaced by scar tissue.

If the infarcted area extends to a serous surface it will produce inflammation of this lining, with fibrinous exudation so that pleurisy is a complication of pulmonary infarction, pericarditis of myocardial infarction, peritonitis of intestinal infarction, and perisplenitis of splenic infarction. In each case, except in the intestine, the inflammation will be followed by the formation of scar tissue and adhesions between the visceral and the overlying parietal membranes. The complication of peritonitis will be mentioned later.

Special Consideration of Infarcts at Individual Sites

The Heart

The softening of the infarcted area may lead to rupture of the wall with the immediate formation of a haemopericardium and death from cardiac tamponade, i.e. the rise in pressure within the pericardium prevents diastolic filling of the heart and results in rapid failure. If a large infarct has healed by scar formation, a cardiac aneurysm may form in the course of time, leading again to the possibility of rupture of the wall.

A common complication of myocardial infarction is the inflammation of the endocardium with the formation of a mural thrombus. Emboli from such a site form the basis of some clinical complications.

The Lungs

Because of the loose texture of the lung and because infarcts of the lung are common when the organs are congested, they are usually haemorrhagic in this situation. It is often difficult at post mortem to determine where an old infarct, which had been clinically obvious in life, existed. This indicates that pulmonary infarcts may resolve and give rise to minimal scar formation.

The Brain

The softening that occurs in infarcts proceeds to liquefaction in the brain so that the end result after the absorption of the fluid is one of cyst formation or a cuplike depression of the surface of the brain if this should be involved.

The Intestine

The peritonitis which complicates infarction of the intestine will not normally heal, because the devitalized bowel quickly becomes infected from the faeces, and generalized peritonitis will ensue unless treatment is given. The infarcted bowel will also lead to the complication of intestinal obstruction.

The Extremities

Infarcts of the extremities arise (i) in old people with severe atherosclerosis of arteries, particularly in diabetics, (ii) in people showing Raynaud's phenomenon due to prolonged arterial spasm, and (iii) in those whose arteries are impacted by large thrombotic emboli. With the exception of Raynaud's phenomenon, the legs are most commonly involved. The ischaemic portion of the limb becomes necrotic and commonly the skin becomes dry, shrunken and blackened (dry gangrene). There is usually a sharp line of demarcation between the dead and viable areas, often with evidence of inflammation at the line of junction. If the infarcted section becomes infected, it putrefies and the lesion is termed moist gangrene.

Congestion

A part is said to be congested when its veins and capillaries are distended with blood (hyperaemia). The congestion can be local or widespread, acute or chronic, active or passive. Active congestion results from arteriolar dilatation with an increased flow of blood through capillaries and veins. Passive congestion occurs when there is venous stasis resulting in diminished vascular flow.

Acute Congestion

The common cause of acute generalized passive congestion is sudden heart failure. In these circumstances the organs will, at post mortem, show a dark purplish discoloration, and blood will exude easily from their cut surfaces. The lungs and the liver are organs where this change is most easily seen. The common cause of acute active, local congestion is acute infection ('rubor'), when, as we have seen earlier, the capillaries dilate and are filled with fast-moving blood.

Chronic Congestion

Local venous congestion occurs if the draining vein is partially occluded. Total occlusion of venous drainage produces venous infarction, whereas minimal occlusion may not lead even to congestion in the affected part if collateral venous drainage is adequate. More generalized venous congestion may be systemic or portal. The cause of *systemic chronic venous congestion* is chronic heart failure. *Portal congestion* follows cirrhosis of the liver or less frequently portal vein thrombosis. Chronic heart failure is most likely to be due to essential hypertension (hypertensive cardiac failure), diffuse pulmonary disease (e.g. emphysema) or to chronic rheumatic heart disease (e.g. mitral stenosis). If the heart failure involves the left side of the heart, the lungs, in addition to the tissues of the rest of the body, show the features of chronic congestion.

Chronically congested *lungs*, when seen at post mortem, are dark red, often with a brown tinge. Blood flows easily from the cut surface, and the texture appears tougher than normal. Microscopically, the capillaries are seen to be tortuous and engorged with blood, some of which will have escaped into the supporting tissues and alveolar lumens. A proportion of the red blood corpuscles will have broken down so that histiocytes containing haemosiderin will be seen in both situations. The characteristic accumulations of these cells in the alveolar lumens are commonly referred to as 'heart failure cells'. The long-standing oedema of the alveolar walls results in fibrosis. The combination of this fibrosis with haemosiderin-staining results in *brown induration* of the lungs. The reduced blood flow through the lungs impairs gaseous exchange and so leads to the important symptom of shortness of breath or dyspnoea, which is a striking feature of congestive cardiac failure.

When the *liver* is the seat of chronic venous congestion it shows a characteristic picture macroscopically, which is often termed 'nutmeg'. The cut surface consists of a regular mosaic of light and dark brown colour, which is due to the difference in response to anoxia of the liver cells surrounding the centrilobular veins, compared with those at the periphery of the liver lobules, adjacent to the portal tracts. The liver cells round the centrilobular vein become degenerate earlier than the peripheral cells because their blood supply is less well oxygenated. The centrilobular cells become necrotic if the venous congestion is relatively acute and severe so that the dark areas in the nutmeg mosaic are due to the distended and congested centrilobular veins and adjacent sinuses, whereas the pale areas are the relatively normal peripheral liver cells. The congestion may be so marked that the dark areas dominate in the mosaic, the pinpoint sized pale zones becoming apparently the centre of dark lobules, a situation which is referred to as 'paradoxical lobulation' of the liver. If the development of the congestion is less acute, the first degenerative features to be seen in the liver cells are those of fatty change. In these circumstances, the earliest picture of venous congestion will consist of fatty liver cells round the congested centrilobular veins with normal cells in the portal zones so that macroscopically the nutmeg mosaic will not be prominent. In the later stages, the centrilobular cells become necrotic whereas the peripheral cells become fatty and thus paler than normal. In these circumstances the mosaic will be much more striking. If the chronic venous congestion is relieved, i.e. by treatment, the structure of the liver returns to normal. If, however, the congestion is both severe and persistent, the necrotic areas do not regenerate but become replaced by fibrous tissue which may link up between adjacent lobules. This relatively uncommon disorganization of liver architecture arising as a result of persistent chronic venous congestion is termed 'cardiac cirrhosis'.

The *spleen* responds in two different ways to chronic venous congestion according to whether it is a result of congestive cardiac failure on the one hand or to cirrhosis of the liver (relatively common) or thrombosis of the splenic vein (relatively rare) on the other. The differences of response are probably due to the fact that the pressure in the portal venous system is much higher and more prolonged in the latter circumstances (portal hypertension) than in the former. In congestive cardiac failure the spleen does not increase much in size, but is much firmer and darker than normal being somewhat inappropriately called a 'cricket-ball' spleen. It cuts very crisply and the cut surface, though very dark, retains its normal markings. Microscopically the bright red of the red pulp contrasts strikingly with the blue islands of lymphoid tissue in the Malpighian corpuscles (or white pulp). With portal hypertension, the spleen enlarges, sometimes to four or five times the normal size, and the capsule may show areas of fibrinous exudate or fibrous thickening. The organ appears somewhat tough on cutting and the cut surface does not show such a marked dark discoloration as in congestive cardiac failure. The splenic pattern is even more marked, however, as a result of thickening of the fibrous trabeculae, and the cut surface may be dotted about with dark areas up to a few millimetres in diameter, which are small haemorrhages resulting from the persistent congestion ('Gandy-Gamna' bodies). Microscopically the spleen of portal hypertension shows a characteristic sponge-like pattern, the widely dilated vascular channels of the red pulp having thicker walls than normal. The fibrous trabeculae are also thicker than normal, and evidence of recurrent small haemorrhages is present, there being foci of siderocytes in the red pulp and impregnation of the fibrous framework with stainable iron as well as foci of more recently shed blood.

Chronic venous congestion of the other organs does not produce striking pathological changes other than a deep purple discoloration due to engorgement of the capillaries and veins. It is, however, not hard to see that this pathological change is the basis of the disorderly function which may arise in these organs as a result of the congestion from reduced blood flow. For example, the patients may have symptoms of indigestion or signs of intestinal dysfunction and the reduced blood flow through the kidneys may lead to oliguria, proteinuria, and cast formation as well as contributing to the formation of the oedema which so often dominates the clinical manifestations of congestive cardiac failure.

5 Hypertrophy, Hyperplasia, Atrophy, Aplasia, Hypoplasia

The weights of most organs do not vary very much under physiological circumstances in any one individual or between one person and another. The organs may, however, respond to alterations in their environment by undergoing hypertrophy or hyperplasia on the one hand or atrophy on the other. *Hypertrophy* of an organ or a cell results in an enlargement to which all the component parts contribute proportionately. *Hyperplasia* of an organ is an enlargement caused not by an increase in size of individual cells but by an increase in their number. There appears to be no fundamental difference between these two ways of enlarging which may in fact often co-exist. Hypertrophy is seen particularly in organs or cells which have lost the ability to divide as for example skeletal muscle. Increase in size is accompanied by RNA synthesis. Hyperplasia is associated with cell division and is accompanied by DNA synthesis. *Atrophy* is the state when an organ or tissue becomes smaller than normal due to a reduction in size or number of its constituent cells. *Aplasia* occurs when a tissue or organ fails to develop and *hypoplasia* when they fail to develop to their full size. The terms aplasia and hypoplasia are also sometimes used loosely for atrophy as in aplastic anaemia. The most certain way of determining whether these changes of size have occurred is by weighing the organs involved.

The exact mechanisms by which these changes of size are brought about are obscure, but certain precipitating factors are recognized.

Factors which cause Hypertrophy and Hyperplasia

1. Response to Increased Work or Need

Response to *work* is seen most clearly in muscular organs. The voluntary muscles of manual workers are larger than those who lead a more sedentary existence. The muscle fibres of the myocardium increase in size if there is increase of resistance distal to the flow of blood. There is, however, no good evidence that the heart gets bigger as a result of continuously increased bodily exercise. The smooth muscle coat of the gastro-intestinal tract increases in size if there is distal obstruction to its lumen. In all these cases, the increase in size is brought about by hypertrophy of individual cells.

Response to *need* occurs when the organs or cells, by metabolizing at their normal rate, are unable to fulfil the functional requirements of the body. For example, if a person has only one kidney either as a congenital anomaly, or because the other has been removed at operation, the kidney will enlarge to about twice the normal size. Red marrow forms blood cells and yellow marrow is inactive in this respect. If there is an increased need for blood cells, such as after a severe haemorrhage, the red cell precursors undergo hyperplasia so that they become more numerous in the red marrow, and may also start to appear in the yellow, with the result that the latter is transformed to red marrow. In chronic renal failure, phosphates may not be excreted as well as they should be, in which case the parathyroid glands increase in size through hyperplasia and secrete more hormone in an attempt to correct the defect in phosphate excretion.

2. Response to Increased Hormone Activity

The anterior pituitary gland provides many examples of this effect. The enlargement of the female breast during pregnancy comes about through a considerable hyperplasia of the lobular acini which later become filled with milk, this increase in size being brought about by prolactin. Enlargement of the thyroid gland also follows the production of an increased amount of thyrotrophic hormone by the anterior pituitary as in puberty or pregnancy. The thyroid cells undergo both hypertrophy and hyperplasia. Bilateral hyperplasia of the adrenals follows increased secretion of corticotrophin and is one of the bases for Cushing's syndrome. Finally, overproduction of growth hormone increases the bulk of most of the tissues in the body, but especially the skeleton. Gigantism results in the adolescent, and acromegaly in the adult.

Increased hormone activity is also probably responsible for other common examples of hypertrophy and hyperplasia. The uterine muscle undergoes considerable hyperplasia in pregnancy. Hyperplastic and hypertrophic changes are a prominent feature of a common abnormality of the female breast called cystic hyperplasia ('chronic mastitis') and also in benign prostatic enlargement, a frequent disorder in the ageing male.

3. Response to Over-nutrition

It might be anticipated that an excessive supply of nutritive materials would lead to an increased size of cells or organs, but apart from the increase in amount of adipose tissue which results from overeating in susceptible individuals, there is no good evidence that this occurs.

Factors which cause Atrophy

1. Response to Under-nutrition

In contrast to the lack of effect of over-nutrition on the size of organs, under-nutrition is an important basis for their atrophy. With persistent starvation, adipose tissue becomes reduced in amount. The size of many of the organs also becomes reduced, though this is least marked in those which are most vital for life, i.e. the heart and brain. The state of replacement fibrosis due to impaired blood supply, and also local atrophy due to pressure, consist of atrophy of parenchymatous cells because of a reduction in the supply of essential nutrients with replacement by less demanding fibrous tissue.

Cachexia also probably comes under this heading, though its mechanism of production is complex and obscure. The term is given to the loss of weight which accompanies certain diseases, particularly malignant neoplasms. This tendency to lose weight varies inexplicably among individuals who apparently have very similar malignant tumours structurally.

2. Reduced Functional Activity

This form of atrophy is most obviously seen in voluntary muscle which has been paralysed for a long time, such as when there has been loss of function of the nerve of supply or when a related joint becomes immobilized. Inactive bone, as in patients confined to bed for a long time, tends to become lighter than normal (osteoporosis). If the normal function of an organ is taken over in part by therapeutic agents, the organ will become atrophic. For instance, blood transfusions given to patients whose marrow can form blood cells well will tend to reduce this normal activity. Again, long continued hormone therapy, for example prednisone, will tend to reduce the size of the organ normally responsible for the production of the hormone which is being given, in this case adrenal cortex. Many organs and tissues undergo atrophy in old persons chiefly because the functional requirements are less, though reduced nutrition and reduced hormone stimulus must also contribute.

3. Reduced Hormone Stimulus

This is best exemplified by reduced functional activity of the anterior pituitary gland. This occurs physiologically on such occasions as at the end of lactation when the breast, which has been secreting milk, returns to its normal size. All the dependent endocrine glands will become atrophic when the whole pituitary gland becomes diseased (panhypopituitarism) or when it is ablated surgically.

Special Features associated with Atrophy

1. Fatty Atrophy

Sometimes when an organ becomes atrophic, the space previously occupied by the erstwhile larger organ is taken up by fat. As already indicated, this occurs in the bone marrow but this fatty atrophy is also a feature of lymph nodes, salivary glands and the thymus when they become atrophic. There is often an increased amount of fatty tissue round the pelvis of the kidney if for any reason the kidney becomes reduced in size.

2. Brown Atrophy

When the cells of some organs become atrophic, they can be seen under the microscope to have accumulated a brown pigment in their cytoplasm, which commonly goes by the name of lipochrome. This change is particularly evident in the heart and the liver, and is reflected macroscopically by the brown colour change which these organs are liable to show in these circumstances.

6 Pathological Effects of Ionizing Radiation

Ionizing radiations occur in two forms, (a) particulate and (b) electromagnetic.

Particulate Radiations

These consist of α-particles, β-particles, neutrons and protons. α-particles are rapidly moving nuclei of helium atoms, which are emitted spontaneously by radioactive elements such as radium and thorium, or are produced by the bombardment of the elements, helium and boron, by neutrons. β-particles are rapidly moving electrons carrying either a negative or a positive (positrons) charge. They are emitted naturally from many radioactive elements, and can also be produced by passing high tension currents through cathode ray tubes. Neutrons are electrically neutral particles which are present in all atoms other than hydrogen. They can be generated in atomic piles from such elements as uranium. Since these particles are electrically neutral they can penetrate the electron cloud of an atom relatively easily and reach its nucleus. The alteration of the nucleus of certain elements which results from this penetration leads to the emission of active ionizing radiations. Protons are the positively charged nuclei of hydrogen atoms which can be accelerated to very high velocities in a cyclotron. α-particles and protons are relatively large and have little penetrating power. β-particles, being smaller, penetrate tissues to a greater, though still limited, distance, i.e. up to two millimetres of tissue. As already indicated, neutrons penetrate relatively easily.

Electromagnetic Radiations

Energy in the form of electromagnetic radiation is produced when an orbiting extranuclear electron passes to a lower orbit. The wavelength of this radiation depends on the energy released, large changes in energy producing very short wavelength γ-rays and smaller changes producing ultraviolet light. X-rays have a slightly longer wavelength than γ-rays. Laser radiation consists of narrow beams of monochromatic light.

The penetrating power of electromagnetic radiation depends on its wavelength. Hence, ultraviolet light has very little penetrating power, whereas γ-rays and X-rays are much more penetrating. Particulate forms of radiation including α-rays and β-rays have very little power of penetration.

Ionizing radiations form part of the normal environment in small and usually harmless amounts. They come in part from the sun (solar or cosmic radiations), in part from traces of radioactive elements incorporated in the soil and in manufactured articles such as bricks. They will also emanate from human bodies themselves—radioactive carbon, for example, exists in bones and its presence there has been used in recent years to estimate the age of those found archaeologically.

X-rays and γ-rays are the forms of ionizing radiation which are most used in clinical practice. β-particles, or electrons, are made use of in certain circumstances, i.e. when radioactive gold or the isotopes of phosphorus and iodine are employed. The radium and radon seeds sometimes inserted into tissues by surgeons are sources of X-rays and γ-rays. The amount of radiation used in X-ray diagnosis is much less than is used in radiotherapy.

The Response of Cells to Ionizing Radiations

When ionizing radiations pass through human tissue they produce ionization in atoms and molecules which lie in their path. Electrons become ejected from some atoms and become attached to near-by ones so that their electric charges become unbalanced. This may cause a disturbance in the molecular pattern leading to a chemical change which in turn may bring about pathological biological effects. Many cytoplasmic enzymes including SH enzymes and adenosine triphosphatase are inactivated by irradiation. The ionizing power of any radioactive source is measured in terms of its effect on a standard quantity of air, and the unit of quantity is a Roentgen (R). The absorbed dose of radiation energy in tissues is expressed in units of rads.

Radiations affect cells most easily when they are undergoing mitosis. Their action has been shown to be more severe when local oxygen tension is high. As with other toxic agents, the harmful effects of ionizing radiations on tissues will depend on the degree of exposure. Very small quantities of radiations such as exist in the atmosphere have no harmful effect, and even the much greater amounts used in X-ray diagnosis, whether in terms of photographic plates or of intravenous radioactive isotopes, such as ^{59}Fe and ^{51}Cr, can safely be given. The harmful effects of ionizing radiations are, however, cumulative which is a good reason for reducing unnecessary exposure to a minimum.

The first biological effect of radiations on cells in mitosis which can be observed is one of temporary inhibition of mitosis followed after an interval of time by an increased rate of mitotic division, i.e. such a dose has a stimulating effect on growth. This effect of X-rays has been made use of clinically in the improvement of eczema of skin. With increased quantities of radiation, cells completely lose their ability to undergo mitotic division, and with higher doses still, necrotic changes can be induced in the mature, non-dividing, cells. When the dose is such that mitotic activity is impaired but the cell remains viable, the visible histological effect is one of enlargement of the cell to a size greater than normal. The shape of nucleus and cell may also become abnormal because of partial derangements of essential cell functions. The visible harmful effects of radiations on cells may take time to appear; the higher the dose, the shorter the time. With doses used in radiotherapy it is not possible to say that an exposed cell, which looks healthy under the microscope, will not develop degenerative changes as a result of the X-rays until three months have elapsed since radiotherapy has been completed.

The tissues of the body vary very much in their sensitivity to a given quantum of radiation. The sensitivity bears a direct relationship to the natural mitotic activity of the component cells. The lymphoreticular tissue, the haemopoietic cells, germinal epithelium, squamous and gastro-intestinal epithelium are the most radiosensitive; the central nervous system and all types of muscle are the most radio-resistant, the remaining tissues occupying an intermediate place (radio-responsive).

As most tissues of the body consist of parenchyma and stroma, the total effect of radiation on the tissue is compounded of the direct action on the parenchyma and indirect action through the effect on the supporting connective tissue. A dose of radiation sufficient to inhibit mitotic activity in epithelium may stimulate fibrous tissue formation and the proliferation of the endothelial cells of the blood vessels. Both the latter effects will indirectly reduce the viability of the epithelial cells.

The response of malignant tissues to radiotherapy varies in the same way as the normal counterparts. However, as the rate of growth, and hence the mitotic activity, are usually above normal, malignant tumours are more sensitive than normal tissues to the effects of ionizing radiations, and this is the basic reason why this form of treatment is given for malignant disease. Another feature of malignant tumours is their tendency to be less well differentiated than the normal cells of the tissues from which they arise; in extreme cases the tumour cells can appear so undifferentiated that it is impossible under the microscope to determine their origin. This lack of differentiation, or anaplasia, is usually accompanied by increased mitotic activity so that undifferentiated tumours are usually more radio-sensitive than well-differentiated forms. However, this increased susceptibility is frequently more than counter-balanced by the increased tendency of the tumour to spread to other situations and so beyond the range of radiotherapeutic control. Another point of difference in response to radiotherapy between malignant and normal cells is that, in the former case, there is frequently a small number in the malignant population which are relatively resistant to the effects of the ionizing radiations. If these survive the first treatment, they multiply and lead to a recurrence of tumour which proves to be more radio-resistant than the original one, and this increased resistance is progressive. It is for this reason that the treatment of many malignant tumours is more palliative than curative.

The Results of Over-Exposure to Radiations

The complications of accidental over-exposure to irradiation will depend on the quantum of incident radiations and the amount of tissues involved. The most frequent risk to over-exposure occurs clinically during radiotherapy, because the margin between the amount of radiation required to kill malignant cells and the amount toxic to normal ones is small. During treatment normal tissue is shielded as much as possible, but inevitably the skin lying over the part irradiated is always subjected to risk of over-exposure. In early stages this may result in hyperaemia and soreness, as in any other type of burn, and a permanent dilatation of the superficial vessels may develop, which can be easily seen through the atrophic epidermis. Later, the combination of the direct and indirect effects of irradiation may lead to a 'radionecrotic' ulcer. The floor of this consists of acellular fibrous tissue in which the capillary blood vessel lumens are practically obliterated by endothelial proliferation and the inflammatory response is less than might be expected. Malignant change in the irradiated skin, i.e. squamous cell carcinoma, is a further possible complication. This was not uncommon in the early days of the clinical use of X-rays, but the greater precautions taken against over-exposure at the present time have considerably diminished this incidence.

Fibrosis is always liable to develop in the deeper tissues when these have had excessive amounts of radiation, and, in certain situations such as the hilar regions of the lungs, may lead to considerable functional embarrassment, such as dyspnoea. Many people feel constitutionally ill after a major course of X-ray therapy, a consequence of the considerable tissue break-down and disorder of normal functions which is the inevitable by-product of such treatment.

Exposure of the whole body to irradiation can take place in different ways. This involves the general public in small amounts all the time, as has already been stated ('background irradiation'). Those handling and conveying radiations as part of their work are at risk to much greater exposure; patients who have to have irradiation over the whole body, as in treatment of malignant lymph nodes, are at greater risk still, and the greatest risk of all, of course, comes to those exposed to nuclear warfare. The effects will depend on the amount and type of radiation received. In the case of atom bombs, the heat of the explosion will kill all close to it. Those farther away tend to die of a generalized illness, 'radiation sickness' presumably resulting from the cessation of vital metabolic activities. Those farther away still may appear normal to begin with, but will eventually decline and die. This appears to be due to the effect on the radio-sensitive reticulo-endothelial system, leading on the one hand to inhibition of antibody production and hence decreased resistance to infection, and on the other to an interference with normal blood formation resulting in aplastic anaemia. Platelet production is often affected earlier than red cell formation so thrombocytopenic purpura may be the earliest manifestation of the aplastic anaemia.

It has been shown that, in a proportion of those surviving exposure to an atomic explosion for some months, there is an increased risk of their developing the malignant disease, chronic myeloid leukaemia. This risk has also been shown to occur in those who are exposed more than normally to other sources of ionizing radiations. For instance, more radiologists have died from this disease than other physicians, and patients who have had a number of X-ray treatments to bones, as in ankylosing spondylitis, also have a higher incidence of the disease. The gonads are also very susceptible to ionizing radiation, with the result that sterility has occurred in those exposed to the hazard. Experimentally it has been shown that the radiations can produce mutations as a result of alteration of genes, and abnormal chromosomes have been shown to occur in chronic myeloid leukaemia and other diseases. This points to the risks of congenital defects developing in the offspring of those people exposed to radiations in doses insufficient to produce sterility.

It is clear, because of the many hazards which arise as a result of exposure to ionizing radiations, that tests should be carried out on those specially at risk in order to see if they are receiving radiations at above a safe level. As the blood cells are early affected by ionizing radiations regular blood counts were for long the means of keeping a check on overdose. It has come to be appreciated that these are not sensitive or exact enough measures and they have been replaced by the wearing of X-ray sensitive photographic plates on coat lapels. This gives a quantitative measure of exposure, which is particularly important as it is known that the ill effects of ionizing radiations are cumulative.

7 Protozoal and Helminthic Infections

Amoebiasis

This is caused by the swallowing of cysts of *Entamoeba histolytica*. The cyst wall is resistant to the acid gastric juices but dissolves in the alkaline intestinal secretion to release the vegetative form. These amoebae may occur in the lumen of the bowel where they do not necessarily give rise to infection, or they may penetrate the mucosa of the large intestine to produce local necrosis and flask-shaped ulcers. Characteristically there is little accompanying inflammation, the necrosis being mostly chemical in nature. The ulcers rarely penetrate the muscle coat of the colon. Amoebae are carried in the portal venous system to the liver where they may cause either a diffuse *amoebic hepatitis* or a local *amoebic abscess*. These abscesses may rupture into the peritoneal cavity, the right pleural cavity or the lung.

Entamoeba histolytica must be distinguished from *Entamoeba coli* which is a gut commensal. *Entamoeba histolytica* in the vegetative form ingests red cells whereas *Entamoeba coli* does not; in the encysted form, *Entamoeba histolytica* has one to four nuclei and *Entamoeba coli* up to eight nuclei. *Entamoeba coli*, being a gut commensal does not penetrate the gut mucosa and so is not found in the tissues in histological sections.

Malaria

This disease occurs most frequently in tropical and subtropical climates. There are four forms of parasite, *Plasmodium vivax* (benign tertian malaria), *P. falciparum* (malignant tertian) *P. malariae* (quartan) and *P. ovale* (similar to benign tertian malaria). The parasites enter the circulation of man by the bite of an infected Anopheles mosquito and there set up the asexual cycle. The introduced *sporozoite* travels to the liver where it remains for seven days, developing into *merozoites*. These are released into the blood stream and enter the red blood cells; here they pass through the developing stages of *trophozoite, schizont* and *merozoite*, which are released by rupture of the red cell to repeat the cycle. The release of the merozoites corresponds with the pyrexial phase—48 hours for tertian and 72 hours for quartan malaria. The sexual phase occurs by some of the merozoites developing into *micro-* (male) and *macro-* (female) *gametocytes*. When the mosquito bites an infected man, these gametocytes are taken with the blood into the mosquito's stomach where they mature to form *gametes*. After fertilization, they form the *zygote* which penetrates the stomach wall to form an *oocyst*. *Sporozoites* develop in the oocyst, now called a *sporocyst*, and rupture of this releases sporozoites into the body cavity of the mosquito. These sporozoites invade the mosquito salivary gland and from there are injected into man to repeat the asexual cycle.

Repeated rupture of red cells may give rise to anaemia, and the phagocytosis of parasites by the reticuloendothelial system results in enlargement of the liver, spleen and lymph nodes. Plugging of the cerebral vessels by parasite-laden red cells may give rise to congestion, small haemorrhages, and focal areas of softening of the brain—*cerebral malaria*. A sudden destruction of red cells may cause haemoglobinuria and jaundice, the latter because the liver is unable to cope with the sudden load of bilirubin resulting from the haemolysis—*blackwater fever*.

Leishmaniasis

Three forms of Leishmaniasis occur. 1. *Cutaneous leishmaniasis*, or *oriental sore*, is caused by *L. tropica*, a round or oval organism, about 2μm in diameter, found particularly in histiocytes in the lesions. It is transferred from a lesion to the new host by a sandfly and causes a skin sore which lasts for weeks or months. The disease is found particularly in the Middle East and Far East. 2. *Mucocutaneous leishmaniasis*. The lesions, which are similar to cutaneous leishmaniasis, affect mucous membranes as well as the skin. The causative organism is *L. braziliensis* and the disease occurs in South

America. 3. *Kala-Azar*, caused by *L. donovani*, is also spread by sandflies. There is proliferation of the reticulo-endothelial system causing hepatosplenomegaly and lymphadenopathy. Phagocytic cells in the bone marrow, lungs, gastrointestinal system, kidneys and skin are numerous and contain many parasites. The disease occurs in Africa and Asia. The massive splenomegaly may be associated with depression of haemopoiesis in the bone marrow resulting in pancytopenia.

Trypanosomiasis

This disease is also known as sleeping sickness. *Trypanosoma gambiense* and *T. rhodesiense* are carried by the tsetse fly. They are slender, flagellate organisms about 15μ in length and up to 3μm in width. The infection causes cerebral oedema, minute haemorrhages and microinfarcts. There is also lymph node hyperplasia and often hepatosplenomegaly. A different variety of trypanosomiasis to that found in Africa occurs in Central and South America (Chagas' disease, caused by *T. cruzi*).

Toxoplasmosis

Toxoplasma gondii, a crescent-shaped protozoon about 5μm in length, causes two types of disease, *congenital toxoplasmosis* associated with transplacental infection and *adult toxoplasmosis*. Congenital toxoplasmosis may result in hydrocephalus, cerebral calcification, choroidoretinitis, pneumonitis and myocarditis. Adult toxoplasmosis causes a disease similar to infectious mononucleosis (glandular fever) but with a negative Paul-Bunnell test. The disease can be confirmed by the characteristic lymph node appearances in which there are focal collections of histiocytes giving rise to granulomata of distinctive appearance. Rarely it may cause pulmonary and cerebral infection in adults. A rising *dye test* titre and *fluorescent antibody* titre are diagnostic of recent infection.

Tapeworms

Man is the definitive host for three types of tapeworm, *Taenia saginata* (beef tapeworm), *T. solium* (pork tapeworm) and *Diphylobothrium latum* (fish tapeworm). The latter is less important in the United Kingdom than the other two worms. Cattle or pigs eat the ova of the tapeworm passed in human faeces. The ova develop into embryos in the animal intestinal tract and these embryos enter the blood stream and become encysted in the tissues. When uncooked, or inadequately cooked meat containing ova is eaten, the ova develop into worms in the human intestine. The head, or scolex, is necessary for the survival of the worm. It is attached to the jejunum by four suckers. The eggs develop in the segments of the worm called proglottids, and these are shed in the faeces. The fish tapeworm is sometimes associated with a megaloblastic anaemia.

Cysticercosis is a disease caused by the ingestion by man of the ova of *T. solium.* These ova hatch in the upper intestine and the larvae penetrate the mucosa to enter the mesenteric vessels. After passing through the lungs, the larvae give rise to systemic infection. Each larva develops into a thin-walled cyst—cysticercus—and there is surrounding inflammation. When the worm dies, the cyst is replaced by dense fibrous tissue and calcification. The brain is a particularly important site for these cysts to form and it is one of the causes of epilepsy.

Hydatid Disease

This disease is caused by infestation by *Echinococcus granulosus* (*T. echinococcus*), the dog tapeworm. The eggs are excreted in the faeces of the dog and are ingested by man, cow, sheep or pig. The eggs hatch in the upper intestine and the embryos penetrate the bowel wall to enter the blood stream. They may be disseminated anywhere in the body. Man may be infected directly in this way or indirectly by eating contaminated meat containing the embryos. When they lodge in the tissues, the common sites being the liver, lung, brain and bone, the embryos develop into hydatid cysts possessing an outer fibrous capsule and an inner germinal layer. From this inner layer, daughter cysts, or 'brood capsules', develop and contain scolices of the young worm. The cycle is completed by a dog eating the tissues from infected animals.

The hydatid cysts may be up to 25 cm in diameter, surrounded by an inflammatory reaction containing many eosinophils. Rupture of the cyst results in secondary cysts and possibly in an anaphylactic reaction. The diagnosis may be established by a positive *complement fixation test* or by cutaneous reaction to the intradermal injection of sterile hydatid fluid (*Casoni test*).

Roundworm

Ascaris lumbricoides are similar to earthworms in appearance. Eggs produced in the human intestine are passed in the faeces. They undergo a period of development in the soil before being ingested. The embryos hatch in the small intestine and pass through the bowel wall into the blood stream. They are carried to the lungs where they set up an allergic pneumonitis. From the lungs they pass up into the major air passages and from there down into the oesophagus to the intestine to complete the cycle.

Hookworm

Ancylostoma duodenale is very much smaller than *Ascaris lumbricoides*, measuring only about 1 cm in length. However each worm can ingest between 0·5 ml and 1 ml of blood each day so that heavy infestation may cause severe iron deficiency anaemia in the host. The ova are passed in the faeces and the embryos hatch in the soil. They gain entrance to the body through the skin and pass to the lungs. From here they pass via the air passages and the oesophagus to the small intestine. The worm attaches itself to the mucosa of the upper small intestine resulting in mucosal oedema and surrounding eosinophilic infiltration. During passage through the lungs, the parasites may cause alveolar haemorrhages and bronchopneumonia.

Threadworm

The ova are deposited around the anus and they are transferred to a new host by faecal contamination. They can frequently be found beneath the fingernails of children. The ova mature in the intestine into adult worms, the male measuring 5 mm and the female 10 mm in length. The commonest symptom is pruritis and caused by the migrating worms depositing ova. Adult worms are frequently seen in appendicectomy specimens, particularly in children.

Trichinella

Trichinella spiralis is a worm measuring up to 5 mm in length. Man is infected most commonly by eating infected, inadequately cooked pork containing encysted larvae. These larvae develop into adult worms in the stomach and upper small intestine. The female penetrates the intestinal mucosa and deposits ova in the submucosa.

The larvae which develop from these ova enter lymphatics and, after passing through the lungs, enter the systemic circulation causing infection of skeletal and cardiac muscle. Initially the larvae cause inflammation of the muscle with many eosinophils but later the larvae become encysted and surrounded by a thick fibrous capsule.

Toxocara

This is a common intestinal worm of cats and dogs being particularly common in puppies. Its importance in man is that the ingested ova develop in the small intestine into larvae which penetrate the mucosa and enter the blood stream. The larvae cause granulomata in the eye and brain and may also give rise to widespread inflammation of the eye leading to blindness. The larvae do not develop into adult worms in man.

Filariasis

This infection is due to *Wuchereria bancrofti,* a thread-like worm measuring up to 10 cm in length. A Culex mosquito takes up the larvae or microfilaria with the blood of an infected patient. The larvae penetrate the gut wall of the mosquito and after undergoing maturation in the thoracic muscles of the mosquito, they pass down the mosquito proboscis to be injected into the skin of man during a further mosquito bite. From the skin, the larvae pass in the lymphatics to the regional lymph nodes and mature in these sites. After mating of the male and female worms, numerous microfilariae are produced by each female. These gain entrance to the blood stream, through the lymphatic channels, the release of microfilariae occurring at night. Death of the worms causes a granulomatous reaction which results in lymphatic obstruction and chronic lymphoedema. The affected parts become grossly enlarged and the skin thickened—*elephantiasis.*

Schistosomiasis

This is the most important infestation due to flukes in man. There are three species of schistosoma, *S. haematobium* (bladder), *S. mansoni* and *S. japonicum* (intestinal and visceral). The eggs are passed in urine or faeces into fresh water, and hatch into larval forms (*miracidia*) which infect fresh-water snails. After a period of development in the snail they emerge as *cerceriae.* These penetrate the human skin during bathing or swimming and enter the blood stream. They pass through the pulmonary circulation and from there enter the portal system where they mature into adult flukes. The parasites lay their eggs in the liver, intestine and bladder where they set up a granulomatous reaction. In the liver this is mainly in the portal tracts and gives rise to a 'pipe-stem' fibrosis. In the bladder there is hyperplasia of the lining mucosa which may progress to carcinoma.

8 Pathological Reactions to Virus Infections

Nature of Viruses

Viruses are intracellular parasites which depend for their metabolic processes upon the host cell. Viruses contain only one type of nucleic acid, either deoxyribonucleic acid (DNA) or ribonucleic acid (RNA) in contrast to all other living cells which possess both. This nucleic acid is surrounded by a protein sheath referred to as a 'capsid' and in some viruses there is a further covering envelope. Virus particles may be arranged in a helical or cubical pattern or a complex of both. The classification of viruses is not universally agreed but a suggested classification is based on the type of viral nucleic acid (DNA or RNA), the presence or absence of an envelope covering the capsid and the geometrical arrangement of the capsids (helical, cubical or complex).

Growth of Viruses

Since they depend on host cells for their metabolic activity, viruses cannot be grown on culture media in the same way as bacteria but require living cells for their propagation. For this reason they are usually grown in tissue culture. The chemical code contained within the nucleic acid of the virus induces the host to synthesize identical molecules of viral nucleic acid and protein from which viral particles are assembled. Viral particles released from damaged cells are adsorbed on to specific sites on the surface of further host cells. This adsorption depends on the specificity of receptors in the protein coat of the virus and it is probable that the predilection of viruses for certain types of cells depends on the specificity of the reaction sites.

Following adsorption, the virus penetrates the cell wall, possibly by phagocytosis, and then is stripped of its outer coverings to reveal the nucleic acid which induces the host to synthesize further viral molecules. These are assembled into viral particles which are released from the cell. This completes the growth cycle of the virus.

Cellular Changes of Viral Infection

Viral damage is most easily seen by their effects on cells in tissue culture, but similar changes occur *in vivo*. The changes produced in cells following viral infection may be described under four headings, *degeneration, fusion, transformation* and *abortive infection*. Degeneration is shown in tissue culture by cells rounding-up, becoming detached from the glass surface on which they are growing, and by the nucleus becoming pyknotic. Inclusion bodies form within the nucleus or cytoplasm. These are intracellular sites of virus synthesis and may be seen in the light microscope, e.g. the intracytoplasmic Guarnieri bodies of vaccinia, the Negri bodies of rabies or the intranuclear inclusions of herpes simplex and chickenpox. Death of the cell may be due to interference with many essential cell functions. Spread of viruses from one cell to another may occur, not by release of viral particles following destruction of host cells, but rather by cell fusion to form multinucleate giant cells or syncytial masses. These are seen not only in tissue culture but also in smears and sections of infected tissues, e.g. herpes simplex and measles.

Some cells after infection with virus do not die but develop new characteristics. They may grow disproportionately in tissue culture, overgrowing other cells, and *in vivo* they may produce tumours. This transformation of cells may be an important cause of some tumours which appear to arise spontaneously in animals but proof of this is still awaited in man. Viruses capable of producing tumours are referred to as *oncogenic viruses*.

Abortive infections arise when the cell fails to synthesize all the molecules required for construction of viral particles. Such cells may show damage, but the virus fails to proliferate within them. This may account for the variation in susceptibility to infection of certain cells and species of animals.

Viral infections initially involve only surface epithelium whether this be in the skin, respiratory, intestinal or urinary tracts or ducts of secretory glands. Many infections remain confined to these surfaces, e.g. warts in the skin, influenza in the respiratory tract. Other infections spread via the vascular system or the cerebro-spinal fluid and these are referred to as sequential infections, e.g. poliomyelitis. These two forms of infection have important clinical significance from the point of view of control of infection.

Immunity Response to Virus Infections

The protein in the virus particles is antigenic and it therefore stimulates antibody production in the host. Both neutralizing antibodies and complement fixing antibodies may be demonstrated in the sera of patients who have been infected. These antibodies do not act on intracellular virus particles and will therefore not be effective against viruses which spread by cell fusion. This explains the latent infection with herpes simplex (cold sore) even when neutralizing antibodies can be demonstrated in the serum. Antibodies are most effective in sequential infections during the viraemic phase. It is in this group that vaccines prepared with inactivated or attenuated viruses are most valuable. They stimulate antibodies which limit the spread of infection. Examples of inactivated viruses used for immunization are poliomyelitis, and examples of attenuated viruses, poliomyelitis, measles and vaccinia.

A low molecular weight protein, *interferon*, produced by cells treated with living or inactivated viruses, inhibits multiplication of viruses. It does not affect extracellular viruses. Passively injected, interferon protects laboratory animals from certain viral infections and this has led to the hope that it may have a role in the treatment of human virus diseases.

Other factors may also play an important part in the body reaction to viral infections and there is evidence to show that cell-mediated immunity contributes to the recovery from infection.

9 The Pathology of the Fluid Compartments

The Normal Composition and Shifts of Body Fluids

1. The Normal Distribution of Fluids and Electrolytes in the Body

The total body water is two-thirds to three-quarters of the total body weight. Approximately two-thirds of the water is intracellular (50 per cent of the body weight). Of the one-third which is extracellular, 20 per cent consists of the blood plasma, the remaining 80 per cent being the interstitial fluid, lying between cells and blood channels. For an adult weighing 11 stones, the total body water is 50 litres, consisting of 36 litres of intracellular fluid, 10·5 litres of interstitial fluid and 3·5 litres of plasma.

The fluid is in a state of constant exchange throughout the body, but the total amount is constant in the normal individual, so that the intake through food and drink will equal the output from the body. An idea of the active movements of the body fluids can be gained from the following table.

Daily Output of Body Secretions

Saliva	1500 ml
Gastric secretions	2500 ml
Bile	500 ml
Pancreatic juice	700 ml
Intestinal secretions	3000 ml
Total secretions	8200 ml

We are quite unconscious of the daily output of this volume of fluid into the alimentary tract, which amounts to more than twice the whole plasma volume, because it is normally all resorbed except for approximately 100 ml excreted in the faeces. The total fluid less from the body in the average normal adult consists of about 2½ litres per day. This takes place in the following way:

Faeces	100 ml
Insensible perspiration	400 ml
Sensible perspiration	200 ml
Respiration	400 ml
Urine	1500 ml
	2600 ml

It will be seen that urine accounts for most of the fluid loss, and it will also be appreciated that it is the main variable, the chief means of adjusting the fluid output under normal circumstances. The 2600 ml of fluid intake which is taken in to match this output is made up in the average person as follows:

Fluids	1450 ml
Water in food	800 ml
Water formed in oxidation of food	350 ml
	2600 ml

Drinking an increased amount of fluid will usually compensate for an increased output, whatever the cause.

The composition of the fluid varies in the different compartments of the body. The chief cation of the intracellular fluid is potassium and the main anions are proteins, organic phosphorus and organic acids. The important cation of the plasma and interstitial fluid is sodium, and the chief anions are chloride, bicarbonate, and in the plasma, proteins. The composition of the fluid in the plasma differs from that in the interstitial fluid mainly in that it contains much more protein, approximately 8 g/100 ml as opposed to 0·1 g/100 ml. The blood vessel wall is relatively impermeable to protein. The intracellular potassium is about twenty-five times as much as that in the interstitial fluid, and the reverse is true for sodium. The potassium and sodium can be regarded as non-diffusible ions, but since the ions can usually pass through artificial membranes easily, their separation by the cell membrane must require expenditure of energy which is probably in most cells supplied through the metabolism of glucose. The anions diffuse across the cell wall more readily, the exchange taking place between chloride and bicarbonate under certain circumstances being called the chloride shift. The exact distribution of fluid in the compartment is proportional to the concentration in them of the non-diffusible ions, like sodium and potassium, and of the non-diffusible colloids like the proteins. The exchange of fluid between plasma and interstitial fluid takes place in the capillaries and through the lymph channels which eventually drain into the thoracic duct.

The factors known to take part in maintaining the flow of fluids and electrolytes between compartments can be summarized as follows:

(i) *The Electrolyte Movement.* The amount of sodium in the extracellular fluid is of paramount importance. If sodium accumulates, water has to be retained as well and this accumulation of extracellular fluid is called *oedema.* Chloride will be the main anion retained. Conversely loss of salt and water from this compartment results in dehydration. Extracellular oedema and dehydration lead eventually to similar changes within the cells. The main factors controlling the levels of sodium and potassium in the body are the food and drink intake and the urinary output. The excretion of sodium and potassium by the kidney is partly mediated by adrenal cortical hormones, especially aldosterone, which enhances the reabsorption of sodium and the excretion of the smaller amounts of potassium. The antidiuretic hormone from the posterior pituitary, by restricting the excretion of water by the kidney, is another important factor in salt and water control.

(ii) *The Hydrostatic Pressure of Blood.* It has been shown experimentally that the capillaries at the base of the nail-bed have blood pressures which vary from 32 mm Hg at the arterial end to 12 mm Hg at the venous end.

(iii) *The Permeability of the Capillaries.* These are permeable to crystalloids and water, but plasma proteins cannot pass freely.

The permeability can be increased by oxygen lack, bacterial toxins, certain poisons and vitamin C deficiency.

(iv) *The Osmotic Pressure of Plasma Proteins.* The high level of plasma protein compared with that of the interstitial fluid produces a difference in osmotic pressure in the two compartments which amounts to 22 mm Hg. The osmotic pressure works in a contrary direction to the hydrostatic pressure, and the plasma albumin is a more important contributor than the globulin partly because its molecule is smaller.

(v) *Lymphatic Drainage.* The flow of lymph into the thoracic duct probably amounts to half a litre per hour under resting conditions.

(vi) *Tissue Tension.* This is higher in some parts of the body than others. For instance in the skin it will be low below the eyes, and high in the palms of the hands. It is particularly low in the alveolar walls of the lungs.

2. The Factors Responding to Sudden Shifts of Plasma Volume

Sudden shifts of plasma volume usually occur in the direction of sudden drops in volume. These will lead, as a result of nervous (vasovagal) reflexes, to a fall in arterial pressure and be accompanied in some individuals by a faint. The fall in arterial pressure is due to a reduction in peripheral arteriolar resistance which most commonly results from loss of blood or plasma to the exterior or the pooling of blood in some part of the peripheral circulation chiefly in the skeletal muscles. The cerebral circulation fails and unconsciousness results. Faints are alarming but not usually serious because of the compensatory mechanisms which come into play. People vary in their tendency to faint because of the variation of the vasovagal reflexes from individual to individual. The fall in arterial pressure promptly leads to modification in the tonic activity of receptor organs situated mainly in the walls of aortic or carotid sinuses. The receptor organs have an effect on cardiac and vasomotor centres in the floor of the fourth ventricle, leading to increase in pulse rate, vasoconstriction in peripheral arteries, and to secretion cf adrenaline and noradrenaline by the adrenal medulla. The effect of these reflexes is to maintain an adequate flow of blood through the vital centres such as the heart and brain.

3. Factors Controlling the pH of the Body Fluids

The pH of the body fluids is kept remarkably constant, between 7·3 and 7·5. A change beyond these limits has a serious effect on health, and the body is able to counter any tendency in these directions by bringing buffering mechanisms into play, and making adjustments back to normal through the excretory activities of the lungs and kidneys.

A *buffer* is a solution of a weak acid and the salt of this acid. The pH does not alter on the addition of relatively large quantities of acid or alkali. This is because weak acids do not ionize very much, i.e. the equation $HA \rightleftharpoons H^+ + A^-$ is very much in the reverse direction. The mixture in the buffer can be written $Na^+ + A^- + HA$.

When strong acid, such as HCl is added, this is equivalent to adding $H^+ + Cl^-$ ions so the mixture in the buffer now reads:

$$Na^+ + A^- + HA + H^+ + Cl^-$$

The $H^+ + A^-$ ions unite to form HA so that we are left with:

$$Na^+ + Cl^- + 2HA,$$

in other words the shift to acidity through the addition of H^+ ions to the mixture has been neutralized by the buffer.

Likewise when a strong alkali such as NaOH is added to a buffer, this means the addition of Na^+ and OH^- ions. The mixture becomes

$$Na^+ + A^- + HA + Na^+ + OH^-,$$

the equation $HA \rightleftharpoons H^+ + A^-$ moves in the forward direction, so the result is

$$2\ Na^+ + 2A^- + H_2O,$$

and the shift to alkalinity is neutralized. The pH of a buffer system such as this can be calculated on the basis of the following equation.

$$pH = K + \log \frac{\text{the concentration of the salt}}{\text{the concentration of the weak acid}}$$

or in short $$pH = K + \log \frac{(NaA)}{(HA)}$$

In the extracellular fluid, the weak acids and salts which are present are H_2CO_3 and $NaHCO_3$, Na H_2PO_4 and Na_2HPO_4, and H Protein and Na Protein. Of these, bicarbonate is quantitatively much the most important, so the pH of the extracellular fluid may fairly be represented by the equation

$$pH = K + \log \frac{(NaHCO_3)}{(H_2CO_3)}$$

If alkali passes into extracellular fluid, carbon dioxide combines with that alkali to form more sodium bicarbonate, and if acid enters the fluid it reacts with sodium bicarbonate to form the sodium salt and carbonic acid. As the effectiveness of this buffer is largely dependent on the quantity of sodium bicarbonate present ($NaHCO_3$), this sodium bicarbonate is called the 'alkali reserve'.

Now the bicarbonate buffering system can obviously operate only with acids stronger than carbonic acid. At times carbonic acid itself will be in excess and another buffering mechanism exists within red cells to deal with this situation; it makes use of the fact that haemoglobin is a weak acid, i.e. the system used consists of $K^+ + Hb^- + HHb$. When excess H_2CO_3 is produced it enters into the red cells with the following result:

$$K^+ + Hb^- + H^+ + HCO_3^- + HHb \rightarrow K^+ + HCO_3^- + 2HHb.$$

By means of the chloride shift mechanism, HCO_3^- passes out of the red cell and Cl^- moves in to take its place, with the result that the bicarbonate in the extracellular fluid, or alkali reserve, increases, but there is no increase in acidity. The red cell buffering mechanism can also come into play in reverse when carbonic acid is lost to the body.

The buffering mechanisms deal with the immediate crisis produced by a sudden increase of acidity or alkalinity in the body. Other mechanisms are also brought into play in the lungs and kidneys, in order to restore the disturbed balance between (HCO_3^- and (H_2CO_3) which has arisen. The lung mechanism comes into operation more quickly. If (H_2CO_3) is increased, then respiratory activity increases and CO_2 is blown off. If (H_2CO_3) is decreased then correspondingly respiration decreases. The kidney makes the more permanent adjustment. The urine contains large amounts of phosphates which form a buffer system, sodium dihydrogen phosphate

(NaH_2PO_4) acting as the weak acid and disodium hydrogen phosphate (Na_2HPO_4) being the sodium salt. This system helps to reduce the alkalinity or acidity of the urine when excess alkalis or acids are excreted. If foreign acid radicles have to be excreted through the glomerular filtrate, sodium ions have to be excreted as well, but these are not lost to the body, because they are reabsorbed by the renal tubules, their place in the urine being taken by hydrogen ions and also ammonium ions formed by the kidney.

Pathological Disturbances of the Composition of the Body Fluids

The pathology of body fluids will be considered under four main headings.

A. Increase of body fluid or oedema.
B. Decrease of body fluid: (i) pure water loss.
(ii) electrolyte loss.
C. Decrease of plasma volume—peripheral circulatory failure.
D. Disturbances of acid-base balance.

1. Oedema

Oedema can be generalized or localized. Special forms of oedema are those which occur in the serous cavities—ascites (peritoneal effusions), and pleural and pericardial effusions. These effusions may or may not be associated with generalized oedema. They are often subdivided into transudates and exudates. Transudates have low specific gravity, do not clot and contain few cells, being non-inflammatory in origin. Exudates arise through inflammation, have a high specific gravity, many cells and clot on standing. The separation on this basis is, however, not always clear cut.

(a) *General Oedema*

(i) *Hypoproteinaemia.* Oedema is liable to occur when the plasma proteins, especially albumin, are low, either as the result of failure to synthesize the proteins or because they are lost from the plasma. Failure to synthesize occurs in starvation and liver disease. Loss occurs through the kidney (proteinuria), especially in the nephrotic syndrome, into the gut (protein losing enteropathy), and through exudation such as in severe burns, in prolonged empyema drainage, or into effusions such as ascites. The low plasma protein level reduces its osmotic pressure so that this is no longer effective in counteracting the hydrostatic pressure of the blood. Hypoalbuminaemia is probably not the only factor in this form of oedema because spontaneous remissions are liable to occur without corresponding alterations in plasma protein levels, and treatment with protein infusions does not always help. The additional mechanisms are still obscure, though in some cases aldosterone appears in excess in the urine.

(ii) *Congestive Oedema.* This arises as a result of cardiac failure. Two factors are known to operate to produce this oedema. Less sodium is excreted by the kidney than normal, and there is increase of hydrostatic pressure at the venous end of the capillaries. The cause of the sodium retention is not yet clear, though excess aldosterone is excreted by the kidney in some cases. It is possible that an intrinsic kidney mechanism also operates. Cardiac oedema has the characteristic distribution of being maximal in the dependent parts. This is because the hydrostatic venous pressure is also at its maximum in these regions.

(iii) *Oedema of Sodium Retention.* This may occur as a result of treatment with adrenal corticosteroids. The most active area of the adrenal cortex concerned with sodium metabolism is the zona glomerulosa which produces aldosterone. Stimulation of the zona glomerulosa occurs through the renin-angiotensin system. A fall in the perfusion pressure of the afferent arteriole of the renal glomerulus results in increased renin production by the juxtaglomerular cells in the vessel wall. Renin, acting on a protein precursor in plasma, produces angiotensin which acts on the adrenal cortex to produce aldosterone. This in its turn causes increased tubular reabsorption of sodium and hence water retention. Normal pregnant women show an increased retention of fluids in late pregnancy and an excess of aldosterone has been found in their urine. The oedema of toxaemia of pregnancy and of glomerulonephritis are largely based on this mechanism.

(b) *Localized Oedema*

(i) *Inflammatory Oedema.* Here, because of the inflammatory reaction, the capillaries become more permeable with the result that fluid passes from the plasma into the interstitial fluid. Plasma proteins leak out in the fluid, as a result of which the interstitial protein level rises, reducing the effective osmotic pressure of the residual plasma proteins thus accentuating the tendency to oedema.

(ii) *Lymphatic Oedema or Lymphoedema.* This is usually to be seen in the limbs and arises in many cases as a result of blockage of lymphatics by tumour cells, inflammation, or parasites. The best-known example of parasitic infection is filariasis. The blockage of lymphatics by this parasite often affects the scrotal skin so that this may become enormously enlarged (elephantiasis). Some cases of lymphoedema are congenital in origin (Milroy's disease), gradually giving rise to subcutaneous fibrosis.

(iii) *Serous Effusions. Pleural effusions* most frequently arise as a result of inflammation, malignant disease or cardiac failure. Effusion may accompany pneumonia, when it may become purulent (empyema). Pleural effusion is a well-recognized presentation of tuberculosis, when it is believed that the capillaries of the pleura become more permeable because of the hypersensitivity which exists in this disease, in addition to being affected directly by the inflammatory reaction to the organism. Malignant effusions are common and arise mainly as a result of the irritation of the pleura by tumour, but sometimes by blockage of the lymphatics. Effusions may be part of the general picture of cardiac oedema, but frequently they are more prominent in one pleural cavity than the other. This difference is brought about by local differences in hydrostatic pressure, produced for example by the kinking of pulmonary veins on one side following enlargement and rotation of the heart.

Pericardial effusions and *ascites* may arise through the same causes as pleural effusions. An important additional cause of ascites is cirrhosis of the liver, and here the mechanism of production is more complex. (1) Hypoproteinaemia leading to reduction of plasma osmotic pressure is common in this disease and arises chiefly because the liver no longer synthesizes albumin efficiently although, if the ascites is continuously drained therapeutically (paracentesis), much protein is also lost in this way. (2) Obstruction to the hepatic venous system by the fibrosis in the liver raises the capillary hydrostatic pressure, so that the interstitial fluid of the liver increases in amount and leaks into the peritoneum. (3) Obstruction to the portal venous system leads to increase of intestinal interstitial fluid, a mechanism which is now not considered to be as important as (2). (4) An increased excretion of aldosterone has been observed in the urine in these cases.

(iv) *Pulmonary Oedema.* This form of oedema occupies a special place because of the urgent clinical symptoms which may arise as a result of the pouring of fluid into the pulmonary alveoli leading to serious respiratory embarrassment and a risk of infection. Pulmonary oedema follows certain forms of cardiac failure, the overloading of the circulation with large volumes of fluid, the inhalation of chemical poisons, cerebral injuries and other rarer causes.

The capillary network is very considerable in the lungs and gets very little mechanical support from the surrounding structures; indeed, in contrast to the normal small positive tissue tension which obtains elsewhere, the respiratory movements exert a negative pressure of 5–10 mm Hg. However, the mean capillary pressure is lower in the lungs than elsewhere varying from 3 mm Hg in the upper parts to 13 mm Hg in the lower. As the plasma osmotic pressure is 22 mm Hg it will be seen that the normal tendency will be for interstitial fluid to move into the capillaries in the upper part, whereas this movement will be less positive in the lower regions. It needs only a little increase in pulmonary capillary pressure for oedema to appear in the lower lobes, though it must be remembered that lymph drainage helps remove some of the excess fluid.

2. Decrease of Body Fluid

A reduced amount of body fluid or dehydration can arise because of (a) pure water loss and (b) electrolyte deficiency.

(a) *Pure Water Loss*

This will arise when for any reason drinking becomes impossible. Examples are lack of access to water, coma, and inability to swallow because of oesophageal obstruction. There is an inevitable loss of a litre a day of water in perspiration and respiration, and of a minimum volume of urine of half a litre. If this loss does not become replaced, the extracellular fluid becomes hypertonic, relieved only slightly by the excretion of salt in the urine. However, water moves from the cells of the body to the extracellular compartment, so that the loss of water is shared, and it will be some time before the volume of body water reaches a dangerously low level.

(b) *Electrolyte Deficiency*

This occurs most frequently through loss of gastro-intestinal secretions, such as in vomiting, diarrhoea, or through fistula formation; it will also result from excretion of salt into the urine, as for example in Addison's disease, where there is loss of the ability of the kidney to conserve sodium. There is loss of sodium as well as chloride from the body during continuous vomiting of acid gastric secretions. This arises because loss of H^+ and Cl^- in the vomit leads to an excess of $Na^+ + HCO_3^-$ in the extracellular fluid. The latter ions are therefore excreted in the urine leading to overall loss of sodium chloride.

When there is a loss of sodium and chloride from the body from any cause, the extracellular fluid volume falls because water is lost as well. Since the extracellular fluid remains isotonic, no water will be drawn from the cells. The natural tendency for people, in replacing this salt and water loss, is to drink fluids low in electrolyte concentration, so the extracellular compartment may then become hypotonic. As a result of this, water will move into the cells, thus augmenting the tendency to a fall in extracellular volume. The kidney will attempt to compensate for the salt loss by excreting a salt-free urine, unless the defect primarily involves this organ. If, however, the salt loss is persistent and unrelieved the volume of the extracellular fluid reaches a dangerously low level, the plasma volume falls, and peripheral circulatory failure will result with renal failure. The latter develops because of the reduced blood flow through the kidney (pre-renal uraemia). As the brunt of the fluid loss will be borne by the extracellular compartment in salt deficiency, dangerous symptoms will arise much earlier than in the case of pure water loss, where the loss is shared with the cells. This effect will be more marked in children than in adults because of the smaller volumes of their body fluids.

While it is convenient to separate the effects of pure water loss and electrolyte loss, it must be remembered that both deficiencies may occur together. This is particularly liable to occur post-operatively.

Salt loss is nearly always a matter of a deficiency of sodium ions, but loss of potassium ions from the body can occur, although a clinically significant reduction is much rarer than with sodium, largely because the total body (intracellular) potassium is much greater than the total body (extracellular) sodium. Potassium deficiency occurs most frequently when there is loss of gastro-intestinal secretions. The deficiency arises because the loss of sodium chloride results in fact in some potassium ions passing the cell membrane barrier into the extracellular compartment, and then into the urine. Potassium loss is likely to be most noticeable after treatment has restored the sodium loss, because potassium then moves back into the cells with a precipitous fall in its extracellular concentration.

3. Decrease of Plasma Volume—Peripheral Circulatory Failure

It has already been mentioned that persistent loss of fluid from the body will lead to peripheral circulatory failure because of a fall in plasma volume. It is appropriate to consider the other important ways by which this fall may be brought about, and to consider briefly the compensatory mechanisms brought into play.

The plasma volume may be reduced suddenly or more gradually. It may occur primarily as a loss of circulating plasma or secondarily as a result of body salt and water deficiency. The causes of the latter have already been given. Sudden reductions of circulating plasma volume occur most frequently as a result of (1) acute haemorrhage when blood is lost to the exterior, (2) 'surgical' shock when, because of the continued nervous stimulation as a result of prolonged surgical manoeuvres, blood is pooled in areas such as voluntary muscles and so is out of circulation, and (3) severe infection, particularly septicaemia, which may produce similar pooling of blood. It will be appreciated that peripheral circulatory failure is particularly likely to occur after severe operations if not corrected by treatment because all three of the above factors could operate. Acute haemorrhage only becomes serious in a previously fit man if he loses 40 per cent of his blood volume or more. Clinical sequelae are minimal if he loses 20 per cent or less, such as when blood is removed for the purpose of donation for blood transfusion. When reduction of plasma volume takes place from any cause, the reflexes mentioned previously (p. 75) are brought into play, as a consequence of which the pulse rate rises and there is an increase of peripheral resistance, both of which mechanisms aid in maintaining an adequate circulation through the vital centres. Eventually, with severe reductions in volume there is a serious decline in cardiac output, a marked drop in blood pressure, a thin and rapid pulse rate, all indicating a failure of the compensatory mechanisms, and death results from failure of the vital organs. Since cerebral cortical cells are more vulnerable to anoxia than the cells of the respiratory and vasomotor centres, loss of consciousness is common before death.

4. Disturbances of Acid-Base Balance

It will be remembered that the pH of extracellular fluids can be represented by the equation

$$pH = K + \log \frac{(NaHCO_3)}{(H_2CO_3)}$$

It will be appreciated from this that alterations of pH could arise primarily as a result of metabolic changes leading to an excess or deficiency of sodium bicarbonate, or primarily as a result of respiratory abnormalities leading to an excess or deficiency of carbon dioxide within the body. The tendency of body fluids to become acid is termed *acidosis*. If the pH lies between 7·4 and 7·3, the acidosis is considered to be compensated; if it is lower than 7·3 it is uncompensated, i.e. the lethal state of *acidaemia* exists. Likewise the tendency of body fluids to become alkaline is termed *alkalosis*. If the pH lies between 7·4 and 7·5 the alkalosis is considered to be compensated; if it is above 7·5 it is uncompensated, i.e. the lethal state of *alkalaemia* exists.

It will be seen from the above that disturbances in the body pH can occur in four ways:

(a) Metabolic acidosis
(b) Metabolic alkalosis
(c) Respiratory acidosis
(d) Respiratory alkalosis

These will be considered in turn.

(a) *Metabolic Acidosis*

The important causes of this state are (1) the over-production of keto-acids as in diabetes mellitus, starvation, and severe dehydration, (2) failure of the kidney to excrete the acid radicles, sulphates and phosphates, which are formed as a result of protein metabolism, (3) excessive therapeutic administration of calcium chloride and ammonium chloride, and (4) loss of base in severe diarrhoea.

The accumulated acids react with the sodium bicarbonate in the extracellular fluid to form carbonic acid. *The* ($NaHCO_3$), *or alkali reserve, thus falls* and reference to the pH equation shows that the pH will fall unless the (H_2CO_3) becomes reduced. This, in fact, takes place through increased respiratory activity, a well-recognized feature of metabolic acidosis ('air hunger'). Uncompensated acidosis will only result if the removal of CO_2 can no longer keep pace with the reduction of the alkali reserve. The kidney, provided it is not primarily at fault as in chronic nephritis, plays its part in restoring the balance in the following way. The excessive amounts of the sodium salt of the keto-acids which have been formed are excreted into the glomerular filtrate. The sodium ions are resorbed in the tubules and their place is taken in the urine by hydrogen and ammonium ions formed by the kidney. Some keto-acids are also excreted direct into the urine. In each event, the acidity of the urine is reduced through the operation of the renal phosphate buffer mechanism (see p. 77).

(b) *Metabolic Alkalosis*

This arises most commonly as a result of vomiting highly acid gastric juice. It can also arise through patients taking too much sodium bicarbonate in order to relieve the pain of a chronic peptic ulcer of stomach or duodenum. The effects of both factors will be to *increase the sodium bicarbonate* (*alkali reserve*) in the extracellular fluid. Reference to the pH equation will show that for the pH to remain steady the body carbonic acid or CO_2 must increase, and if and when this increase becomes inadequate, the dangerous state of alkalaemia will result. The increase of carbonic acid is achieved by lowering of the respiratory rate which reduces the loss of CO_2 through the lungs. The excess of sodium bicarbonate which has been formed is excreted through the kidney and the resulting alkalinity of the urine is reduced by the phosphate buffering mechanism which is brought into play. In the late stages of the alkalosis produced by excessive vomiting the overall deficit of extracellular sodium may become so great that all the sodium bicarbonate is resorbed by the tubules. This results in the excretion of an acid urine, even though a state of alkalosis exists.

(c) *Respiratory Acidosis*

This arises because there is some obstruction to the normal expiration of carbon dioxide in the lungs. It is most likely to arise as a result of mechanical obstruction of respiratory passages as in emphysema or pulmonary fibrosis or because the respiratory rate has been suppressed, i.e. as a result of excess of morphine therapy. The effect is an accumulation of carbonic acid in the body. Reference to the pH equation will show that if the pH is to remain normal, *the* ($NaHCO_3$) *or alkali reserve must rise.* Acidaemia will result only when the body can no longer add more sodium bicarbonate to the extracellular fluid. The red cell buffering mechanism is brought into play to produce this increase of sodium bicarbonate (see p. 77).

(d) *Respiratory Alkalosis*

This is the least common of the disturbances of acid–base balance. It can be brought about by overbreathing, either deliberate or hysterical, or may occur following injury to the brain after such episodes as road accidents. Carbon dioxide is washed out to excess in the lungs reducing the extracellular (H_2CO_3). Reference to the pH equation shows that in order to maintain the pH at a normal level, *the* ($NaHCO_3$) *or alkali reserve must fall.* Alkalaemia will result only if the ($NaHCO_3$) fall can no longer keep pace with the (H_2CO_3) fall. The red cell buffer mechanism is important in reducing the amount of extracellular ($NaHCO_3$), though excretion of the bicarbonate by the kidney plays its part.

It will be seen from the above descriptions that the alkali reserve will be low in metabolic acidosis and respiratory alkalosis, whereas it will be increased in metabolic alkalosis and respiratory acidosis. Clinical confusion between the metabolic and respiratory causes of disturbed acid–base balance is highly unlikely, and it is because of this state of affairs, and the fact that metabolic disturbances are clinically much more frequent than respiratory ones, that the lowering of the alkali reserve is commonly accepted as a yard-stick for acidosis, and an increase for alkalosis. The pH can only be worked out on the basis of the pH equation precisely if the concentration of dissolved carbon dioxide in the body fluids is known. This is an estimation much more difficult to carry out than the measurement of the alkali reserve.

10 | Allergy, Anaphylaxis Autoimmunity, Collagen Diseases

It has already been seen in Chapter 2, that when an antigen gains access to the body, it stimulates the production of antibodies which play an essential role in eliminating that antigen. An example of such a reaction is bacterial infection where the antibodies eliminate an organism and give rise to a state of immunity to further infection. Immunity falls into two main categories, humoral and cell-mediated. Humoral immunity is associated with circulating immunoglobulins produced by plasma cells in response to soluble or particulate antigen which can be transported to lymph nodes and spleen. Cell-mediated immunity is found when antigen is fixed in tissues such as tissue homografts. Under these circumstances, small lymphocytes passing through the antigenic tissue are sensitized. They are transported to regional lymph nodes where they proliferate in the paracortical area to give rise to large lymphocytes, or immunologically active cells. These cells eventually return to the antigenic tissue with which they react. This cell-mediated immunity is known to be thymus dependent in early foetal life. Removal of the thymus in experimental neonatal animals causes a failure of cell mediated immunity and a state of tolerance to foreign antigens.

Hypersensitivity Reactions

An unexpectedly vigorous response to antigenic stimulation is referred to as *hypersensitivity* or *allergy*. Four types of hypersensitivity are recognized; the first three are associated with humoral antibodies and give *immediate type hypersensitivity* and the fourth is associated with a cell-mediated response and gives *delayed type hypersensitivity*.

Immediate Type Hypersensitivity

Type I

The term anaphylaxis is given to the acute immunological reaction which sometimes develops on the post-primary inoculation of antigen or hapten. This anaphylactic reaction can occur in a generalized fashion or involve a local area only, depending on the degree of sensitivity of the individual, the site of introduction of the antigen and on the dose of antigen. The generalized anaphylactic reaction is usually severe and constitutes a clinical emergency liable to result in death. The phenomenon occurs widely in the animal kingdom, some animals being more susceptible than others and each species having its distinctive clinical syndrome. In man the anaphylactic state produces bronchospasm, hypotension, tachycardia and shock. There may be angioneurotic oedema of the skin, laryngeal oedema, conjunctivitis, diarrhoea and vomiting. The reaction is caused by antigen combining with reaginic antibody (IgE) formed from previous exposure to the antigen, and fixed to the surface of mast cells. The antigen-antibody reaction causes rupture of mast cells which release histamine, 5-hydroxytryptamine, plasma kinins and slow-reacting substance. The latter, produced mainly in the lung, is a powerful stimulant of smooth muscle and accounts for much of the bronchospasm. This type of reaction can be transmitted in serum and is seen in the *Prausnitz-Küstner reaction*—if serum containing reaginic antibody is injected into the skin of a normal individual followed by pricking of antigen into the sensitized site, it produces a local reaction of an anaphylactoid pattern.

Type II

This form of hypersensitivity develops when an antigen forms part of a cell membrane or basement membrane. Complement is usually required to produce cell damage. Such a pattern of reaction is seen in haemolytic disease of the newborn. In this condition a mother of Rhesus negative blood group is sensitized usually by foetal Rhesus positive cells entering her circulation. Previous blood transfusions may also sensitize. Antibodies form in the mother and these antibodies may cross the placenta in future pregnancies to react with Rhesus positive antigen on the surface of foetal red blood cells causing haemolysis.

Type III

When soluble antigen and antibody react they may produce an immune complex which is precipitated in vessel walls. Complement is activated and this attracts polymorph leucocytes which further damage vessel walls causing an acute vasculitis. Such a reaction is the basis of the *Arthus phenomenon.* The subcutaneous injection of non-toxic antigen initially causes no response, but injections repeated at weekly intervals cause progressively more severe local vascular damage. This is due to the reaction of antibody within vessels reacting with antigen outside the vessels to form a precipitate in the vessel wall. Arthus sensitivity may involve sites other than the skin. Inhalation of dust containing thermophilic actinomycetes found in hay, results in Arthus sensitivity in the lungs, giving rise to the condition of farmer's lung and leading to pulmonary fibrosis.

Serum sickness is another cause of Type III hypersensitivity. In this condition, antigen stimulates antibody production, and this antibody then reacts with antigen still present in the tissues. Some of the antibody may be IgE and give rise to anaphylactic (Type I) hypersensitivity, but if IgG antibody is formed this will complex with the antigen and give rise to myocarditis, arthritis, glomerulonephritis and arteritis.

Delayed Type Hypersensitivity

Type IV

This is cell mediated and does not depend upon the presence of humoral antibodies. In sensitized individuals the reaction is maximal 24–48 hours after exposure to the antigen and is characterized by a perivascular cuff of mononuclear cells, most of which are lymphocytes with fewer macrophages. Examples of delayed type hypersensitivity are found in the Mantoux reaction in which protein purified derivative of tuberculin (PPD) is injected intradermally. There is no reaction in a normal person, but in one who has had a tuberculous infection it produces local erythema and oedema 24–48 hours after the injection.

Theories of Antibody Formation

There are two principal theories concerning immune responses whether these are humoral or cellular. The first theory referred to as the *instructive* theory postulates that antigen enters immunologically active cells and acts either as a template for the formation of antibody or modifies the nucleic acid to synthesize antibody. The second or *selective* theory is now based largely on the clonal hypothesis of Burnet. In this theory it is postulated that immunologically active cells exist, capable of reacting with antigenic groupings. When these cells are exposed to antigen they proliferate to form a clone of cells which can react specifically either by producing humoral antibody to that particular antigen or can take part in specific cell-mediated reactions. If antigen is present in great excess it kills off the specific immunologically active cells so that a state of tolerance is induced. It is possibly by such a process that antigens belonging to the host (self antigens) are not rejected throughout life for the cells capable of producing an antibody reaction would have been killed during intrauterine life. In such a way the body comes to recognize proteins as *self* or *non-self*. The role of the thymus in cell-mediated immunity has already been mentioned (p. 87). Removal of the thymus in early neonatal life of young animals causes depletion of lymphocytes in the paracortical region of lymph nodes and the periarteriolar white pulp in the spleen—*thymus dependent areas*. It is these cells which are capable of proliferating to cause cell-mediated immunity. Their depletion results in a state of tolerance to grafts of foreign tissue.

Autoimmunity

For many years it was believed that the body was incapable of producing antibodies to its own tissues but more recently it has come to be appreciated that under certain conditions this is not so. Diseases are now recognized in which antibodies directed against host tissues may be demonstrated in the patient's serum, giving rise to a state of autoimmunity. It is important to appreciate that the demonstration of autoantibodies in the serum is not always accompanied by tissue damage. Further, autoantibodies may result from tissue damage due to other factors and may not contribute to the disease. Caution must always be exercised before attributing a disease to autoimmunity. Where a disease may reasonably be called autoimmune, the tissue damage is often the result of cell-mediated rather than humoral immunity. Various factors must now be considered to explain the failure of recognition of self and non-self antigens.

Development of Autoantibodies

New tissue antigens may be produced at a stage after the development of immunological maturation. During foetal life, according to the selective theory of antibody formation, cells which are capable of reacting with 'self' antigens are destroyed. However, sex cells develop in later life so that if they come in contact with immunologically competent cells they may not be recognized as 'self' and antibodies may be produced against them. If a tissue does not normally come in contact with antibody-forming cells, as for example the uveal tract, it will not have been recognized as 'self' in early life. Later exposure, as follows damage to the eye, may result in an immunological reaction directed against the cells of the uveal tract leading to the condition of sympathetic ophthalmia.

A failure of the immunological mechanism may result in the release of 'forbidden clones' of cells capable of damaging 'self' tissues. It has been postulated that the thymus is important in the formation or removal of 'forbidden clones' and this may account for the thymic hyperplasia or neoplasm that accompanies autoimmune diseases such as myasthenia gravis. Cell mutation resulting in lymphoid neoplasms, lymphatic leukaemia and malignant lymphomas, is another possible mechanism for the formation of cells capable of reacting against 'self' antigens. Autoimmune haemolytic anaemia and thrombocytopenia are common in patients with lymphoid neoplasms. Host antigens may be altered by infections or by physical or chemical agents and so may not be recognized as 'self'. An example of physical agents altering host antigens is cold. Exposure to cold in susceptible individuals leads to urticaria. Chemical agents may form a hapten link with host protein altering its antigenicity and making the protein autoantigenic. At other times, antibodies may be directed against the chemical agent rather than the hapten-linked protein, and as such the antibodies are not strictly autoantibodies. Viral infections may also alter tissue antigenicity. If mice are infected with lymphocytic choriomeningitis (LCM) virus before immunological maturity they have a transient illness but then recover in spite of widespread viral particles in many tissues. However, if the mice are infected with LCM virus after immunological maturity they develop a fatal illness with lymphocytic infiltration of infected organs. The illness therefore appears to be due to an immunological reaction damaging the tissues and not due to the virus itself. It is possible that other viral infections, e.g. mumps, may produce damage by a similar mechanism. If homologous antigen, e.g. brain, is injected in Freund's adjuvant (an oil-in-water emulsion of killed tubercle bacilli) it produces an enhanced immunological reaction and autoantibodies are formed. A similar mechanism of enhanced response may account for the autoantibodies found in tuberculosis, leprosy and syphilis. Wasserman antibody used in the diagnosis of syphilis is an example of such an autoantibody. Patients with these diseases may also have rheumatoid factor, antinuclear factor and thyroid autoantibodies in their serum.

Lastly there may be a cross reaction between foreign antigens and host antigens. A possible example of this is seen with Group A haemolytic streptococci which have in their coat an antigen very similar to that in sarcolemma of cardiac muscle and smooth muscle of blood vessels. There is a well-known clinical association between this organism and rheumatic fever which is characterized by damage to the heart with the formation of Aschoff nodes. Although antibodies to cardiac muscle can be demonstrated in the serum of about half the patients with rheumatic fever, no immunoglobulins have been demonstrated in the Aschoff nodes. The reaction may therefore be cell-mediated or the cardiac damage may be due to the direct toxic action of the infecting organism.

It will be seen that there are many ways in which autoimmune disease may develop. However, the temptation to place diseases of unknown aetiology into this category without critical analysis must be resisted.

Collagen Diseases

With the recession, as a result of antibiotics, of the frequency of bacterial infections as a cause of fever, it came to be appreciated that this symptom was sometimes due to one of a group of disorders which could well be called sterile inflammations. The tissue changes had a common factor in that foci of connective tissue developed a staining reaction resembling fibrin and referred to as 'fibrinoid degeneration'. These 'collagen diseases' include systemic lupus erythematosus, dermatomyositis, systemic sclerosis (scleroderma), polyarteritis nodosa, rheumatoid arthritis and rheumatic fever.

Systemic Lupus Erythematosus

One of the diagnostic features of this disease is the LE cell. This is a polymorph leucocyte which has engulfed a homogeneous basophilic body consisting of denatured nucleo-protein. LE cells are produced by the action of a serum factor on nuclei, the denatured nuclei then being taken up by polymorphs. The serum factor is an immunoglobulin (IgG) which can react against host nuclei (antinuclear factor or ANF). It is now believed that free DNA escapes into the circulation of these patients possibly due to the presence of an inhibitor of an enzyme (DNAase) which normally removes any free DNA. The circulating DNA reacts with antinuclear factor to form precipitates of immune complexes which are removed in the kidneys, heart, joints and in vessels in other tissues. It has been demonstrated that these precipitates not only contain DNA but also IgG, complement and fibrin. The disease is very similar to a spontaneous disease occurring in NZB mice which develop haemolytic anaemia, hepatosplenomegaly and glomerulonephritis. It has been shown recently that these mice have a congenital viral infection. It could well be that this virus causes the release of DNA into the serum resulting in an autoimmune disease. In spite of the similarity of SLE and the mouse disease, the aetiology of SLE remains uncertain.

The commonest lesions in lupus erythematosus are in the kidney, spleen, heart and skin. In the kidney, there is a proliferative glomerulonephritis with deposition of immunoglobulins in the basement membrane of the glomerular capillaries to give 'wire loop' thickening of the membrane. The renal arteries commonly show a vasculitis with fibrinoid necrosis. There is also a vasculitis in the spleen and in the heart with a pericarditis. The endocardium may be affected, giving rise to small vegetations on the valve cusps (Libman-Sacks endocarditis). Light-exposed areas of the skin show erythematous inflammation. On the face this may have a 'butterfly' distribution over the nose and cheeks.

Dermatomyositis

This is a disease of adults and about 20 per cent of cases have an associated neoplasm. There is an erythematous rash and muscle weakness. Occasionally antibodies are formed in the serum which react with tumour extracts and immunoglobulins can be demonstrated in the skin and muscle.

Systemic Sclerosis

This is associated with thickening of the dermis and fibrosis of many organs including the alimentary tract, heart and lungs. There may be an arthritis, glomerulonephritis and vasculitis. About 80 per cent of these patients have antinuclear factor in their serum. A similar disease may be produced in experimental animals by injecting homologous lymphocytes into recipients previously made tolerant, producing a graft versus host reaction in about three weeks.

Rheumatoid Arthritis

This disease consists predominantly of chronic inflammation of synovial joints. There are also subcutaneous nodules which occur around joints and in sites exposed to trauma. The nodules consist of foci of fibrinoid necrosis surrounded by palisaded histiocytes, lymphocytes and plasma cells. The joints show villous hyperplasia of the synovium, which is more vascular than normal and heavily infiltrated by lymphocytes and plasma cells. The proliferating synovium spreads over the articular cartilage to form a 'pannus' which may result in fibrous ankylosis of the joint. Granulomatous lesions may also be found in the heart and lungs. The serum of most of these patients contains 'rheumatoid factor' which is demonstrated by the Rose-Waaler test. In this test patient's serum is used to agglutinate sheep red blood cells coated with a rabbit anti-sheep cell antibody. This rheumatoid factor is now identified as an IgM immunoglobulin and the antigen with which it reacts is IgG. The cause of the disease is still largely speculative. It shows features similar to those of Reiter's syndrome, in which there is urethritis, arthritis and uveitis. Reiter's syndrome is believed to be due to infection with a mycoplasma. A disease similar to rheumatoid arthritis can be produced in animals simply by injecting Freund's adjuvant (an oil-in-water emulsion of dead tubercle bacilli).

Rheumatic Fever

Although this disease usually follows infection with a β haemolytic streptococcus, these organisms cannot be isolated from rheumatic lesions. It has already been seen (p. 92) that these streptococci have an antigen in their coat very similar to that found in the sarcolemma of cardiac muscle and the smooth muscle of blood vessels. The illness usually develops when antibodies are forming. The classical inflammatory focus in the myocardium is the Aschoff node. This involves the interstitial connective tissue of the heart and consists of fibrinoid necrosis surrounded by characteristic mesenchymal cells (*Anitschkow myocytes*) and lymphocytes. Multinucleate giant cells are also found; these are smaller than Langhans giant cells found in tuberculosis. Identical lesions may be produced in rabbits by the repeated intravenous injection of foreign protein. Although the heart is the principal organ involved, the joints and brain (chorea) may also be affected.

Polyarteritis Nodosa is described on p. 153.

The concept of collagen diseases is useful and it has helped in that it has focused attention on a group of diseases with many similar signs and features of altered immunological response. It should not be taken to mean that they have a common aetiology nor that they have a similar pathogenesis.

Further Reading

Turk, J. L. (1969) *Immunology in Clinical Medicine.* London: Heinemann.

11 Gene and Chromosome Pathology

Chromosomes

During cell division, nuclear chromatin gathers together to form threads called *chromosomes* each of which splits lengthwise to form two *chromatids* joined at one point called the *centromere*. Chromosomes are composed of basic proteins, histones, and deoxyribonucleic acid (DNA). Information about the appearance of chromosomes has accumulated recently due to improved methods of tissue culture. The addition of colchicine to the culture causes arrest of cell division in metaphase so that dividing cells accumulate and their chromosomes can be studied in stained preparations. Under these circumstances the two arms of the chromatids separate, being held only by the centromere, to form the shape of the letter X. The size of the chromosomes and the position of the centromere, whether it is central or towards one pole, is constant for any particular chromosome. In the human there are 46 chromosomes made up of 22 pairs of *autosomes* and two sex chromosomes. In the male these sex chromosomes are referred to as X and Y whereas in the female there are two X chromosomes. According to the characteristics of the chromosomes they can be arrayed in 7 groups referred to as a *karyotype*. Germ cells, i.e. ova and spermatazoa, are different from somatic cells in that they have only half the number of chromosomes, i.e. 23. The nuclei of somatic cells are called *diploid* and those of the sex cells *haploid*. If nuclei have many more than the usual number of chromosomes such as happens with many malignant cells, they are called *polyploid*.

In normal females, a condensation of chromatin, called the *Barr body*, can be found adjacent to the inner aspect of the nuclear membrane. Barr bodies are not found in normal males. The number of Barr bodies is one fewer than the number of X chromosomes. It has been suggested that this is because only one X chromosome is active and the other is condensed and inactive. Similar sex chromatin can be seen in polymorph leucocytes as a 'drum-stick' appendage to the nucleus. Nuclei containing sex chromatin are referred to as *chromatin positive* and those without as *chromatin negative*.

Cell Division

There are two forms of cell division, *mitosis* and *meiosis*. The two chromatids held together at the centromere in the early stage of mitotic division eventually separate at the centromere and move to opposite poles of the cell where they form daughter nuclei. This is followed by constriction of the cytoplasm so that two daughter cells form with the same number of chromosomes as the parent cell. The germ cell precursors undergo meiotic or reduction division, which consists of two stages. In the first stage, pairs of chromosomes come to lie alongside one another. At points along each chromosome they seem to be attached to the corresponding site on the partner. It is apparently at these points that cross-over of the chromosomes occurs with exchange of chromatin material from one chromosome to another. Each chromosome then separates from its partner and they gather together to form two daughter nuclei which immediately pass into the second stage of division which is comparable with mitotic division. The result of the full meiotic division results in four haploid nuclei. All the male cells survive as spermatozoa but only one of the four female cells survives as an ovum. When conception takes place the spermatozoon unites with the ovum, so the newly produced cell, or zygote, will have 46 chromosomes, one of each of the 23 pairs coming from the father, and the other from the mother.

Gene Abnormality

Genes occupy a specific place on the chromosome. As the chromosomes consist of identical pairs, it follows there will also be gene pairs. The gene occupying a certain place on a chromosome is not always precisely the same; it may be one of a small group of possibilities. These groups of possible genes to occupy a single locus in a chromosome are called *allelomorphs*. Groups of genes controlling certain characteristics tend to be inherited together (linked genes), i.e. they move together in the crossing over which takes place in meiosis. The majority of genes cannot be assigned definite sites on chromosomes but a few have been assigned to the X chromosome (sex-linked genes), the best known being those controlling haemophilia and colour blindness. Genes possess varying grades of potency from complete *dominance* to complete *recessiveness*. This phenomenon is important when considering the behaviour of gene pairs. If the bearer has both genes dominant or both recessive, he is termed *homozygous* with respect to the gene; if one gene is dominant and the other recessive, he is *heterozygous*. Occasionally an individual gene will undergo some sudden alteration of behaviour and, presumably, of structure, which results in its determining a new and distinctive character in its bearer. When this happens, *mutation* is said to have occurred.

Any inherited gene which determines a character seriously detrimental to the health or life of the bearer is liable to lead to his premature death. The gene is thus likely to be eliminated from the population by operation of natural selection. This is most likely to occur if either one or both of a pair of genes is dominant, because so many of the second generation are likely to have inherited the gene and therefore the abnormal character. This elimination by natural selection is much less likely to occur if the abnormal genes are recessive, because the disease itself will only appear in those individuals who are homozygous for the affected gene. This type of individual can only be born to parents, both of whom have the abnormal gene.

The diseases recognized to be examples of dominant inheritance are very rare, the best known perhaps being neurofibromatosis or von Recklinghausen's disease, polyposis coli, and one of the types of progressive muscular dystrophy. Other muscle diseases are examples of recessive inheritance, as is a well-known but uncommon skin abnormality, xeroderma pigmentosa. Haemophilia is the best-known disease due to a sex-linked recessive gene. Since the gene is attached to the X chromosome, it becomes obvious in males, but in heterozygous females it is masked by the dominant partner gene on the corresponding paired chromosome. Females are therefore symptomless carriers except for the very rare homozygous haemophiliac female.

Chromosomal Abnormalities

Abnormalities in the karyotype may be either numerical or structural. Numerical abnormalities may result from failure of pairs of chromosomes to separate during meiosis (*non-disjunction*), resulting in both chromosomes being included in one nucleus, with a resulting deficiency in the other nucleus. Tetraploid cells may result from failure of separation of chromosomes so that they are all enclosed by a single nuclear membrane. Structural abnormalities result from breaking of the chromosome with irregular rejoining of the broken fragments. This may result in *translocation* of chromatin material from one chromosome to another, or *deletion*, with loss of chromatin material. Since genes occupy a specific place on chromosomes and groups of genes controlling certain characteristics tend to be inherited together (linked genes), it follows that abnormalities of chromosomes will result in corresponding abnormalities of genetic structure.

Sex Chromosome Abnormalities

Klinefelter's syndrome is characterized by a male phenotype but usually possesses chromatin-positive nuclei due to an additional X chromosome giving a total of 47 chromosomes and XXY sex chromosomes. Clinically these patients have atrophic testes, infertility, eunuchoidism and mental defect. ***Turner's syndrome.*** In contrast to Klinefelter's syndrome, these patients are of female phenotype but are chromatin negative. The most common chromosome pattern is 45 with loss of one of the X chromosomes. These patients show sexual infantilism, webbing of the neck and cubitus valgus. There may also be other congenital defects.

Autosomal Abnormalities

One of the most important is Down's syndrome (mongolism) occurring in 1 in 700 births and due to autosomal trisomy. Patients show severe mental retardation with typical physical characteristics of epicanthic folds, flat nasal bridge, protruding tongue, flattened occiput, transverse palmar crease and incurving little finger. The incidence of the disease increases with advancing maternal age to 1 in 50 and this is now believed to be due to increasing risk of non-disjunction of the 21 chromosome during meiotic division to form the ovum. The syndrome can also be produced by translocation of the 21 chromosome to another chromosome, usually 15. Translocations of this pattern may be identified in a carrier mother indicating the considerable risk of further affected children.

Autosomal abnormalities have been detected in cells of patients with malignant disease. Polyploidy has been demonstrated in malignant tumour cells and is one factor responsible for the hyperchromatism which is such a characteristic histological feature of malignant tumours. A chromosome with a missing arm, known as the *Philadelphia chromosome*, is a constant abnormality in chronic myeloid leukaemia. It is of interest that it is the same chromosome which is abnormal in Down's syndrome where there is an increased risk of *acute* leukaemia.

Congenital Abnormalities

Registered infant mortality from malformations has remained constant numbering 5 per 1000 births since the beginning of the century whereas the total infant mortality has dropped from 130 to 20. The malformations which thus are assuming increasing importance consist mainly of such changes as anencephaly, spina bifida, hydrocephalus, cardiac abnormalities, hare lip and cleft palate, defective limbs, pyloric stenosis and Down's syndrome. Down's syndrome is the only one of the abnormalities which is known to be purely genetically determined. Environmental factors are clearly important in other cases, for example the drug thalidomide leads to defective limb development, and there is an increased risk of congenital defects following maternal rubella infection. Ionizing radiation may also lead to chromosomal abnormality. It is possible that most congenital abnormalities will be found to be due to a mixture of genetic and environmental factors, but this is at present a speculation which might, however, be resolved by further studies in cytogenetics.

Further Reading

Carter, C. O. (1969) *An ABC of Medical Genetics.* London: Lancet.

12 Neoplasms (New Growths)

A *neoplasm or new growth* consists of a mass of cells which have undergone some fundamental and irreversible modification in their physiology leading to their continuous and apparently unrestrained proliferation. A neoplasm is often referred to as a *tumour*, although strictly the latter word merely indicates the presence of a swelling, which could be due to other causes such as inflammation or cyst formation. *Cancer* (Latin: a crab) is probably the word used most often by the layman for a neoplasm, although the tacit assumption is that cancer is one of the more sinister variants which will extend crab-wise into the surrounding tissues. Any cells in the body can give rise to neoplasms, although the transformation occurs more frequently with some than others. The cells which do not undergo replacement or regenerate under normal circumstances, i.e. nerve cells or voluntary muscle fibres, are the ones least likely to produce neoplastic counterparts. Neoplasms usually involve one type of cell principally but a number exist in which two or more cell lines take part. The change from a normal to a neoplastic cell appears to take place suddenly and permanently, so that the neoplastic cell transmits its new qualities to its descendants, giving rise to a mass of tissue independent of the cell of origin. This sudden transformation has all the qualities of a genetic mutation and the probability that this is what happens is supported by the fact that many cancer cells have been shown to have an increased number of chromosomes (polyploidy). The cause of this sudden change is the key to the cause of cancer and is still largely unknown despite a great deal of investigation. However, a considerable amount of relevant information has accumulated, which will be summarized in a later chapter.

Neoplasms usually start at one site in the body, but there are some, chiefly those developing in lymphoid tissue (e.g. lymphosarcoma), which may arise in different parts of the body at the same time (multicentric origin). The rate of growth of neoplasms varies a great deal, some taking many years to expand, slowly compressing the adjacent tissue to form a surrounding fibrous capsule and showing no evidence of increased mitotic activity of its component cells, whereas others show appreciable change in their size within a few days with a large number of often abnormal mitotic figures in the component cells, and with extension far beyond the confines of the original abnormality. These two extremes in behaviour of tumours form the basis of their being classified into *benign* and *malignant* forms. The slow expansile growth of benign tumours will usually cause little inconvenience to their hosts, unless the swelling leads to compression of a near-by vital structure, such as the brain, with interference to its function, or unless the tumour is one of secretory cellls, producing an excess of the secretion concerned. An example of the latter is the rare islet cell tumour of the pancreas which may produce an excess of insulin and lead to hypoglycaemic symptoms. The fundamental difference between malignant and benign tumours is that, left to themselves, the malignant tumours will grow more quickly and extend deeply and widely into the surrounding tissue at many points so that no capsule forms between them and the neighbouring tissue, and in the course of time they will appear in other situations in the body forming secondary masses of tumour (*metastases*). Unless the growth of malignant tumours is controlled early on by surgical or other means of treatment the unrestrained cell multiplication will eventually so seriously interfere in one way or other with normal bodily functions that death will inevitably ensue. Indeed the eradication of the undesirable effects of malignant tumours is one of the major problems of clinical medicine, for of the half a million deaths that occurred in England and Wales in 1969 over a hundred thousand, or one-fifth of the total, were due to this cause.

When neoplasms are examined microscopically, a wide range of cell pictures will be encountered. Benign neoplasms tend to reproduce very faithfully the cells of their normal counterparts which are grouped together with ancillary structures such as blood vessels and nerves just as they would be in normal tissues. As has been pointed out, mitotic figures are uncommon, and often, but not invariably, a fibrous capsule will separate the tumour mass from the surrounding normal cells. Even when no capsule exists there is in most cases a clear line of demarcation between the tumour and its environment.

Malignant tumours show a much wider range of cell patterns than benign ones. At one extreme they will look very similar to the tissues from which they arise; at the other the resemblance will have disappeared completely. When the tumours exhibit the former pattern they are termed *well differentiated* and when the latter, *poorly differentiated* or *anaplastic*. Even when well differentiated, the malignant tumours tend to show a number of features which distinguish them from normal tissues. The cells are usually not so tidily knit together to form the tissues they give rise to as normal ones. They also tend to show a wider range of variation in size both of cytoplasm and nucleus (*pleomorphism*). More than one nucleus may be formed in an individual cell, and there is a tendency for the nucleus-cytoplasm size ratio to become greater than in the normal cell. The nuclei themselves are usually darker than normal (*hyperchromatic*), frequently because they contain an increased number of abnormal chromosomes. Mitotic figures are more numerous and may include many bizarre forms. Because of the disorderly and rapid growth of malignant tumours, they do not develop a satisfactory blood supply in the way that benign ones do; in fact the tumour cells often rely on the existing blood vessels of the host tissues. These are frequently insufficient to supply the nourishment required by the tumour cells so that degeneration or necrosis is a frequent occurrence in malignant neoplasms. The line of demarcation between malignant tumours and the tissues from which they arise is usually not clear. Some, however, grow in expansile fashion to begin with so that they tend to form capsules, but the line of cleavage is rarely as clear as in benign tumours. More often clumps of malignant tumour cells are seen *infiltrating* between the cells of the normal surrounding tissues so that the two elements are inextricably bound together. The malignant tumour cells move along the lines of least resistance. The precise reason for this behaviour is unknown. However, it has been shown that, while malignant cells have no distinctive properties when seen under the electron microscope, they adhere less firmly to each other than normal ones, and some tumours have also been shown to produce a hyaluronidase-like enzyme which is capable of softening the stroma round the tumour cells.

As has been pointed out a distinctive property of malignant tumours is their ability to reach other parts of the body, and to grow to form *secondary tumours* or *metastases* there. There are three main routes by which they achieve this: (1) by way of lymphatics, (2) by way of blood stream and (3) across serous cavities (pleura, peritoneum, pericardium). The factors which influence the development of metastases are still largely unknown, though it is clear local factors are important because secondary tumours form more commonly in some organs than others. Evidence, largely based on a study of the spread of malignant melanomas of the skin, has recently accumulated which indicates that humoral and cellular antibodies are formed by the host which limit the primary tumour and restrict the growth of metastases. The cellular reaction around many malignant tumours may have a similar role. Rapidly growing melanomas show a deficiency of the host immune reaction.

(i) *Lymphatic Spread.* Tumour cells have the property of being able to infiltrate through the thin-walled lymphatic channels in their neighbourhood, and then either grow along the lymphatics (permeation) or be carried along by the lymph to the lymph nodes into which the lymphatics drain (embolization). Microscopically the first evidence that tumour cells have arrived in a lymph node is the appearance of a small clump at the periphery in the cortical sinus. If the tumour cells are able to continue to grow, they usually do so within the sinuses at first, but eventually they will completely replace all the lymphoid tissue of the node, and even extend beyond the confines of the capsule of the node. The lymph nodes in this way temporarily hold up the progress of the malignant tumour, and this is the basis for one of the standard surgical treatments of malignant disease, viz. block dissection of the regional lymph nodes. However, the malignant cells frequently pass on from one lymph node to another and it is not an uncommon clinical experience to find a metastasis in a lymph node which is remote from the site of origin. Sometimes neoplastic cells will spread along lymph channels in retrograde fashion because the normal drainage area has been blocked by the formation of lymph node metastases: this is an explanation for metastases being observed in unexpected places. The malignant cells may find their way eventually into the thoracic duct and thus be disseminated widely in the body by way of the blood stream. Tumour may also spread by way of perineural spaces, which is quite a frequent phenomenon, and is probably the cause of the development of pain in many instances.

(ii) *Blood Stream Spread.* The arterial wall is relatively resistant to infiltration by malignant neoplasms, which gain access to the blood stream more frequently by way of the veins or capillaries. When the tumour cells penetrate through the endothelial lining of these vessels they are liable to become the nidus for thrombus formation, and the fragmentation of these malignant thrombi is the starting point of some of the blood-borne metastases, but free circulation of individual malignant cells undoubtedly occurs as well. The malignant cells are carried along in the venous system either through the right side of the heart to the lung capillaries or, if they start within the alimentary tract, through the portal vein to the sinusoids of the liver. Most of these tumour emboli die at their point of impact, some proliferate to form metastases, and others permeate along the capillary walls to reach the wider channels distally whence they disseminate. In the case of the lungs this is by way of the systemic arteries and so to all parts of the body; in the case of the liver it will first be into the hepatic vein and the inferior vena cava and thence through the right side of the heart to the lungs.

(iii) *Transcoelomic Spread.* Once a malignant tumour has infiltrated through the endothelial surface of the serous cavities of the body it is liable to appear in the form of secondary nodules elsewhere in that cavity. These nodules may be few in number or be so numerous as to form a practically continuous lining over the membrane surface. It is considered by most that this 'transcoelomic' spread occurs because tumour cells fragment from their site of original penetration into the cavity and subsequently seed themselves elsewhere on the membrane surface. There are some, however, who consider that spread by way of the lymphatic network beneath the membrane surface plays an important part in the dissemination of the tumour. This development of secondary tumours in the walls of serous cavities is quite a common event, especially within the peritoneum and the pleural cavity. The tumours usually lead to the formation of fluid exudates, and the cytological identification of malignant cells in the aspirated fluid is often of great diagnostic help. In the peritoneal cavity, the ovaries are particularly prone to become the seat of secondary tumours (Krukenberg tumours).

As a rule, neither benign nor malignant tumours contribute anything to the body's economy, i.e. they are entirely parasitic. They are little subject to laws governing normal growth, i.e. they live an independent existence or are *autonomous*. However, both are capable of reproducing some of the activities of normal cells, such as secretion of hormones, which in extreme cases may provide symptoms attributable to oversecretion.

Table I summarizes the features which distinguish benign tumours from malignant ones.

TABLE I

Benign	*Malignant*
Remain localized	Can form metastases
Slow growth	More rapid growth
Often has a capsule	Capsules rare and incomplete
Mitotic figures rare	Mitotic figures frequent
Very similar to cells of origin	Less similar, and in some cases totally undifferentiated
Cells of uniform size and appearance	Cells and nuclei vary in size and shape, and nuclei often hyperchromatic
Degenerative changes relatively uncommon	Degenerative changes relatively common

Just as no essential difference in structure has been identified between malignant and normal cells, so no metabolites have been found exclusive to malignant cells. The chemical composition of malignant cells differs quantitatively but not qualitatively from normal ones. Little also is known of enzyme substrate system differences, though what is known suggests that differences here might provide the clue as to why malignant cells are so autonomous in their behaviour.

A striking effect of some malignant tumours on the host is their ability to cause considerable loss of weight, and a sense of malaise, a syndrome usually referred to as *cachexia*. Malignant tumours are unpredictable in their ability to produce cachectic states, some small ones having an unexpectedly pronounced effect while some large ones may be ineffective in this respect, at any rate till the later stages. Further, of two tumours of identical size and apparently similar morphology in different patients, one may produce considerable cachexia, and the other very little. There is clearly competition by the tumour in cachectic patients for nutrient substances, especially nitrogenous ones needed for the host's metabolism, but the details of this competition remain largely obscure.

Malignant tumours are occasionally associated with other, little understood, syndromes. These include a flitting form of venous thrombosis (thrombophlebitis migrans) seen particularly in association with pancreatic carcinoma, demyelination of nerve tracts of the central nervous system in the absence of metastatic tumour in the area, muscle weakness which resembles a primary muscle wasting (myopathy), dermatomyositis, and the skin condition, acanthosis nigricans.

Finally it must be emphasized that distinction between new growths on the one hand and other conditions which give rise to tissue hyperplasia or proliferation on the other is in practice by no means always easy. The most helpful criterion in reaching a decision as to whether new formed tissue is a true tumour or not is the fact that neoplastic proliferation involves a fundamental cellular change and is an automatic process so that, once it has started, it is independent of the continued presence of the initially provocative agent, whereas other hyperplastic masses will cease to grow and even regress on withdrawal of the stimulus producing the hyperplasia.

Further Reading

Evans, R. W. (1966) *Histological Appearance of Tumours.* 2nd edn. Edinburgh, Livingstone.

Willis, R. A. (1952) *The Spread of Tumours in the Human Body.* London, Butterworth.

Willis, R. A. (1967) *Pathology of Tumours.* 4th edn. London, Butterworth.

13 Nomenclature and Classification of Neoplasms

No nomenclature of neoplasms is universally accepted because no system has yet been devised which is completely satisfactory. Various systems have been proposed of which the *histogenetic classification* based on the type of tissue from which the tumour has arisen is the most widely used. The primary division into *behaviour pattern* of benign and malignant forms has been discussed in the previous chapter. The *shape* of the tumour is commonly used in classification. This is sometimes of value for the prognosis depends to some extent on the pattern of tumour growth, whether in a solid plaque or in frond-like outgrowths. The *site of origin* of the tumour, is clearly important, but it is necessary to combine a classification based on this with a histogenetic classification, for tumours occurring in a particular organ may be arising from widely different tissues. Classifications based on *embryological origin* of the tissue are of limited value but classification based on *aetiology* may become more important as our understanding of the aetiology of neoplasms increases. At present it is too limited to form a worthwhile classification.

The terminology followed here is one based mainly on histogenesis. Where more than one name is commonly used for any one tumour, both will be given. The basis for division depends on whether the component cells have arisen from epithelium, connective tissue including haemopoietic and lymphoreticular tissues, nervous system or a group of tumours derived from a mixture of tissues. A few tumours do not fall into any of these categories.

A. Epithelial Neoplasms

Descriptive terms indicating structural features are frequently used, the two most common in this connection being *papilloma* and *polyp*. The papilloma consists of a frond-like outgrowth of neoplasm on an epithelial surface. The term polyp is used for any pedunculated mass arising from an epithelial surface and is not necessarily neoplastic. Many polyps have an inflammatory cause.

1. Benign Epithelial Tumours

The nomenclature is based on the type of epithelium concerned, whether it is stratified or simple in its make up or whether it arises from an organ or viscus showing either internal or external secretory activity. The stratified epithelium consists of two main structural types—squamous and transitional epithelium.

Squamous Cell Papillomas

These are most commonly seen on the skin surface where they are often called warts. They are good examples of the way in which it is difficult to distinguish clearly between true neoplasms and other forms of hyperplasia. Many of the warts which form on the skin are in fact due to virus infection, and will disappear when the virus is no longer active, so that, although they look neoplastic, they are examples of focal hyperplasia.

Transitional Cell Papillomas

These are most frequently seen in the urinary bladder, but may arise anywhere where transitional epithelium normally exists, i.e. the renal pelvis and the ureters.

Adenomas

Adenomas are tumours arising in secretory epithelium. They may project from an epithelial surface or grow in the substance of glandular tissues. The former are common in the large intestine where they are either papillary adenomas or adenomatous polyps. Among the best-known solid adenomas are those arising in the thyroid. Sometimes adenomas are largely cystic in their make up, with papillomatous projections into their cavity. A good example of this type is the papillary serous cystadenoma of ovary.

2. Malignant Epithelial Tumours

These are called *carcinomas* (or carcinomata), and are subdivided in a similar way to their benign counterparts.

Squamous Cell Carcinoma

This name is given to the tumour which shows some evidence of maturing in the same way as normal skin, i.e. prickle-cells develop and the most mature cells become keratinized. However, because of the tumour's infiltrating properties, the relation of the cells to the surface becomes lost, with the result that the tendency to keratin production is liable to occur in the centre of a clump of tumour cells deep in the tissue ('cell nests' or 'horny pearls'). The tumour arises at sites normally lined by stratified squamous epithelium, for example the skin, lips, buccal cavity, pharynx, oesophagus, larynx and the cervix uteri. A commonly used, but not well-chosen, synonym for the neoplasm is 'epithelioma', particularly when it arises on the skin or lips. Squamous cell carcinoma may also develop at sites not normally lined by stratified squamous epithelium. For this to occur, the normal epithelium usually undergoes a change, most commonly from a glandular to a stratified squamous epithelial pattern (*metaplasia*) and the latter then becomes neoplastic, but occasionally this pattern of carcinoma can arise without preceding metaplasia. The best-known example of a metaplastic carcinoma is in the bronchus where it accounts for about half of all the carcinomas, and is the type which is most prone to arise in heavy smokers. Other sites for this metaplastic phenomenon are urinary bladder, renal pelvis, and gall-bladder. In the last two instances the presence of calculi in the cavities is a common association.

Squamous cell carcinomas show a tendency to metastasize by way of lymph nodes before the blood stream.

Basal Cell Carcinoma

This tumour is another carcinoma arising from stratified squamous epithelium but having distinctive qualities. It is usually found on the skin, most commonly on the face. It may form a solid mass of cells, in which case it tends to remain localized for a long time, or it may form thin columns or trabeculae when it shows a much more invasive quality. The former variety is closely allied to congenital abnormalities of skin or naevi. The latter is the form which has given the tumour its synonym 'rodent ulcer'. If not successfully treated, the carcinoma will ulcerate the skin producing the characteristic circumscribed ulcer with raised, smooth, grey edges, and will excavate the underlying tissues of the face producing disfiguring cavities. A feature of all varieties of basal cell carcinomas is that they do not metastasize. Histologically, the tumour pattern is characteristic, consisting of hyperchromatic small cells similar to those in the basal layer of the skin, showing little variation in size. The bigger cell masses frequently develop a distinct palisade of regularly arranged basal cells at the periphery.

Transitional Cell Carcinoma

These tumours develop, like their benign counterparts, most frequently in the urinary bladder but also in the renal pelvis and ureter. Transitional cell tumours show such a great tendency to recur when removed and to infiltrate the underlying wall that a lower histological threshold for the diagnosis of carcinoma exists here than anywhere else in the body. The diagnosis is made, even if the transitional epithelium shows only slightly greater hyperplasia than normal, with minimal variation in cell size. This means that in hospital practice transitional cell carcinomas are much more common than papillomas. The carcinomas can take either papillary or solid forms; the former carry a better prognosis than the latter. Lymph node and blood stream spread are relatively infrequent, largely because the pathological changes in the renal tract, i.e. infection or uraemia, often lead to the death of the patient.

Adenocarcinomas

Adenocarcinomas are malignant tumours which arise from secretory or glandular epithelium, and therefore exist widely in the body. Among the commonest are those of the gastro-intestinal tract, but breast, kidney, ovary, prostate, thyroid, pancreas and biliary passages are other tissues which are not infrequently implicated. The particular features of the tumours of the individual sites will be described later. The better differentiated adenocarcinomas resemble quite closely the normal epithelium from which they are derived but will usually, even then, show some atypical features, such as disorder of arrangement of cells, failure of secretory activity, variation of cell size and evidence of infiltration. All carcinomas, but particularly adenocarcinomas, excite differences in stromal reaction by the host. At one extreme the fibrous stroma is so abundant that the malignant cells may be hard to identify within it; at the other there is so little fibrous reaction that the tumour consists chiefly of solid masses or alveoli of malignant cells. The hardness of a carcinoma observed clinically is proportional to the amount of fibrous tissue present. When it is abundant, the tumour is often referred to as being 'scirrhous', when scanty 'encephaloid'.

Most adenocarcinomas arising from glandular surface epithelium or secretory glands, metastasize primarily by way of lymphatics and later by the blood stream. However there are exceptions to this rule, and adenocarcinomas derived from mesenchymal organs such as the kidney metastasize more frequently by way of the blood stream. Transcoelomic spread is important for adenocarcinomas arising in the gastro-intestinal tract and ovaries.

Undifferentiated Carcinomas

A proportion of carcinomas when examined under the microscope will be so undifferentiated that it is impossible histologically to say whether they are squamous, transitional or adenocarcinomas. They are then referred to as undifferentiated or anaplastic carcinomas. When this situation arises, the carcinoma is usually more malignant and metastases tend to occur early, so that the prognosis for the patient is poor. Some carcinomas are so anaplastic that it becomes very difficult to determine whether they are carcinomas or other forms of malignant disease. If the undifferentiated cells tend to exist in solid masses or columns, separated by newly formed fibrous tissue, they are likely to be carcinomatous.

B. Connective Tissue Tumours

Although it is convenient to think of connective tissue cells as being of specific type, such as cartilage cells, fibroblasts or fat cells, metaplasia of one type of cell to another occurs with great ease. For this reason tumours of connective tissue often show many types of tumour cells. It is customary to classify these tumours according to the predominant tumour cell or to the most malignant component where several tissues are mixed.

The names given to the benign tumours of connective tissue consist of the suffix *-oma* combined with the prefix indicating the tissue of origin. The tumours involving cells of the lymphoreticular and haemopoietic systems do not follow this general rule for no benign tumour of this group is known to exist with any certainty and no uniformity of opinion exists as to the nomenclature of the malignant counterparts. Probably the most acceptable and widely used terms are *myeloproliferative disorders* for the neoplasms primarily involving cells of the bone marrow and *malignant lymphomas* for those primarily involving lymphoid tissue. 'Reticulosis' is a commonly used synonym for the latter.

The names given to the malignant tumours of connective tissue are called *sarcomas*, and similar prefixes to those used for their benign counterparts are applied when it can be certain that these malignant tumours arise from the corresponding tissues. The poorly differentiated sarcomas are usually described according to the shape of the predominant cell, i.e. spindle-cell, round-cell or polygonal-cell sarcoma.

Lists of the main members of the whole group of connective tissue tumours follow.

(a) General List

	Benign	*Malignant*
Fibrous tissue	Fibroma	Fibrosarcoma
	(Myxoma)	(Myxosarcoma)
Fatty tissue	Lipoma	Liposarcoma
Bone	Osteoma	Osteosarcoma
Cartilage	Chondroma	Chondrosarcoma
Smooth muscle	Leiomyoma	Leiomyosarcoma
Striated muscle	Rhabdomyoma	Rhabdomyosarcoma
Blood vessels	Haemangioma	Haemangiosarcoma
Lymphatics	Lymphangioma	Lymphangiosarcoma
Synovium	Benign synovioma	Synovial sarcoma
Mesothelium		Mesothelioma

(b) Neoplasms of the Lympho-reticular System

(i) *Myeloproliferative disorders*
Chronic myeloid leukaemia
Chronic lymphatic leukaemia
Myelomonocytic leukaemia
Acute leukaemia
Polycythaemia vera
Thrombocythaemia
Erythraemia
Myelofibrosis
Myelomatosis

(ii) *Malignant lymphoma*
Lymphocytic lymphoma
Lymphoblastic lymphosarcoma
Histiocytic lymphoma } (Reticulum
Stem cell lymphoma } cell sarcoma)
Hodgkin's disease

Thymoma

1. Benign Connective Tissue Tumours

These are extremely common but most go undetected during life as they do not produce clinical symptoms. One of the commonest tumours is the *leiomyoma* arising from smooth muscle in the uterus. These tumours may be multiple and give massive uterine enlargement. With time they gradually become replaced by fibrous tissue and so they are often referred to as uterine fibroids. They may eventually calcify.

Most *fibromas* arise from nerve sheaths and are referred to as neurofibromas. A fibrous tumour arising in the dermis of the skin, dermatofibroma, is less well defined than most benign tumours and there is still debate whether to regard it as a true neoplasm or reactive hyperplasia. Fibromas may be found in the ovary. Some of these at least, represent the end stages of tumours either derived from the theca around ovarian follicles (thecoma) or they are mixed tumours consisting of islands of epithelium in a fibrous stroma (Brenner tumour).

Occasionally fibrous tumours occurring in fascial planes have a mucinous consistency. This may be so marked as to mimic Wharton's jelly in the umbilical cord, hence the term *myxoma*. As with more typical fibromas many of these tumours are derived from nerve sheaths.

Lipomas are common tumours found most often in subcutaneous fat giving a smooth, lobulated swelling. They are often multiple and consist of mature adipose tissue.

The term *osteoma* is often given to the reactive new bone at sites of chronic irritation, e.g. overlying chronically inflamed frontal sinuses or beneath the big-toe nail, or the term may be used for bony excrescences. The term is more appropriately used for distinctive tumours occurring in the long bones referred to as *osteoid osteoma.*

Chondromas can be single or multiple, the latter being dubiously true neoplasms, as they are frequently associated with congenital abnormalities. Such tumour-like malformations are called *hamartomas*. Chondromas may grow in the centre of a bone (enchondroma) or they may grow outwards (ecchondroma). They commonly occur in the long bones, including the metacarpals and phalanges. Ecchondromas may ossify to give *exostoses*, erroneously referred to as *cancellous osteomas.*

Most so-called *haemangiomas* are in fact congential aberrations of growth (e.g. port-wine naevi). If a tumour consists of close-packed capillary blood vessels, it is termed a capillary haemangioma; if it is made up of vessels with wider lumina and smooth muscle fibres in the walls, it is termed a cavernous haemangioma. A skin nodule consisting of proliferating granulation tissue referred to as a *granuloma pyogenicum* may easily be confused with a haemangioma.

Lymphangiomas, like haemangiomas, are common. They are distinguished by the nature of the contents of the neoplastic vessels. Lymphatic swellings consisting of thin walled lymphatic vessels containing lymph are developmental malformations, e.g. the *cystic hygroma* which develops in the neck of infants.

Tumours of striated muscle are extremely rare. So-called *rhabdomyomas* are hamartomas found in cardiac muscle in association with tuberose sclerosis.

Benign synoviomas occur as small brown nodules on the tendon sheath usually in the hand. Many regard these as being reactive hyperplasia of synovium.

2. Malignant Connective Tissue Tumours

These are less common than their benign counterpart. As with all malignant tumours they are poorly circumscribed, infiltrating surrounding structures. They invade vascular channels, but unlike carcinomas, they metastasize predominantly by way of the blood stream to the lungs; lymphatic spread is much less common.

Fibrosarcomas occur mainly in the soft tissues of the limbs and retroperitoneum but they may also arise from bone, either from the periosteum or from the sheath of nerves supplying the bone. In the dermis of the skin, *dermatofibrosarcoma protuberans* is a locally infiltrating fibrous tumour which tends to recur after excision but which characteristically does not metastasize. Mucinous or myxomatous change is common in soft tissue fibrosarcomas, especially those derived from nerve sheaths. When the myxomatous change is so great as to form a jelly-like mass, these fibrosarcomas may be referred to as *myxosarcomas*. They are more liable to recurrence after excision because they are less clearly defined and, following operation, tumour cells spilt into the wound may grow to form a fresh tumour.

Leiomyosarcomas most commonly arise from the smooth muscle of the gut or from the uterus. Their behaviour is notoriously difficult to assess histologically and often the mitotic activity is a better guide to their malignancy than is cellular pleomorphism.

Liposarcomas are uncommon tumours. The better differentiated show evidence of their origin in fat; those that are less well differentiated may show many tumour giant cells. In these tumours, small droplets of fat do not offer proof of origin in adipose tissue, for fat may occur in a variety of tumours as a degenerative process.

Osteosarcomas are rare tumours which occur mainly in adolescents and young adults, arising towards the ends of the long bones, especially around the knee. In older people, osteosarcomas may arise as a complication of Paget's disease of bone. These are highly malignant tumours with very few five-year survivals. Because of the poor prognosis, it is important to identify the true nature of these tumours. They often possess other elements such as fibrous tissue and cartilage but the formation of bone matrix, osteoid, by the malignant tissue is the essential diagnostic feature.

Chondrosarcomas arise in the same sites as osteosarcomas, and although they metastasize by way of the blood stream to the lungs, they do so less readily than osteosarcomas.

Rhabdomyosarcomas are very rare. Two patterns are seen, those arising in infancy and childhood and those arising in old age. The infantile embryonal rhabdomyosarcoma arises in sites such as the orbit, oropharynx, bladder, prostate and vagina whereas the adult variety arises in the main bulk of skeletal muscle. Both are highly malignant neoplasms.

Angiosarcomas, whether derived from blood vessels or lymphatics, are highly malignant tumours. Lymphangiosarcomas sometimes arise in patients with long-standing lymphatic obstruction due either to a congenital abnormality (Milroy's disease) or following irradiation of the axillary lymph nodes for metastatic breast carcinoma. *Kaposi's sarcoma* is a rare tumour consisting of proliferating blood vessels and spindle cells which occurs in the skin and internal organs. It is still debated whether it should be regarded as an angiosarcoma.

Synovial sarcomas occur in the large joints or in bursae in fascial planes. They mimic normal synovium by forming clefts resembling joint spaces. These are lined by epithelioid cells but elsewhere the tumour consists of spindle cells.

Mesotheliomas arise from the pleura and peritoneum. There is a close association between these tumours and inhalation of asbestos dust (asbestosis).

The malignant tumours of the lymphoreticular system are more appropriately described in the section on systematic pathology.

C. Neoplasms of the Nervous System

As these tumours form a heterogeneous group, it is convenient to divide them up into the following types:

NEOPLASMS OF THE NERVOUS SYSTEM

Brain and spinal cord	Glioma
Meninges	Meningioma
Adrenal medulla and sympathetic chain	Ganglioneuroma
	Neuroblastoma
	Phaeochromocytoma
Nervous fibrous tissue	Neurofibroma
	Neurofibrosarcoma
	Neurilemmoma
Melanoblasts	Juvenile melanoma
	Malignant melanoma

All these tissues are of neuro-ectodermal origin. In the brain and spinal cord, tumours of neurones are very rare as these cells have a very limited capacity to divide. Most of the primary tumours are therefore derived from the neuroglia and fall into three groups, *astrocytoma*, *oligodendroglioma* and *ependymoma*. *Medulloblastomas* are also usually classified as gliomas because of their behaviour but they are derived from cells which have not differentiated into neurones or neuroglia. They metastasize in the cerebrospinal fluid but very rarely outside the nervous system. The most malignant gliomas infiltrate and are rapidly growing. The less rapidly growing may be classified as 'benign' but their behaviour may be far from benign due to pressure and involvement of vital centres.

Tumours of neurones are more common outside the central nervous system and then arise particularly in the adrenal medulla and retina. The *neuroblastoma* of the adrenal medulla is a malignant tumour of young children that metastasizes by the blood stream to bones. *Retinoblastomas* are histologically similar tumours but they are less malignant. *Ganglioneuromas* consist of mature neurones and their supporting cells and fibres. There is good evidence to show that these benign tumours form by maturation of neuroblastomas.

Meningiomas are firm tumours which arise from the meninges usually in the parasagittal region and along the wing of the sphenoid. They compress the underlying brain and although they are 'benign' they may eventually infiltrate neighbouring structures.

Phaeochromocytoma is a tumour which arises in the adrenal medulla from cells which have an affinity for chrome salts (chromaffin). The tumour secretes adrenaline and noradrenaline and may give rise to hypertension.

Neurofibromas and *neurilemmomas* are derived from Schwann cells of the nerve sheath. Neurofibromas are usually multiple and appear to arise by expansion of the whole nerve bundle. They are less well defined than neurilemmomas which are usually solitary and often occur in the skin. An *acoustic neuroma* is a neurilemmoma arising on the eighth cranial nerve. Neurofibromatosis (von Recklinghausen's disease) is a familial disease with dominant inheritance in which many neurofibromas and neurilemmomas occur. Transformation to neurofibrosarcoma is more likely to occur with the larger deep-seated tumours.

Tumours which involve the cells which produce the brown pigment melanin (melanoblasts) are also described here, because most people believe that these cells take origin from the neural crest and migrate from there in embryonic life to their final positions, chiefly in the skin. The most common swellings due to collections of these cells are the pigmented lesions in the skin called *cellular naevi* or *moles*, which are sometimes warty, and sometimes merely flat discolorations. These moles are not true tumours but congenital malformations. They are liable however to undergo malignant change, forming *malignant melanomas*. Cutaneous malignant melanomas are usually considered to have a very bad prognosis because of the ease with which they metastasize but this is not always the case with early lesions. The neoplasm spreads both to the regional lymph nodes and to other situations in the body by way of the blood stream. Another important site where malignant melanomas arise is the eye. Here, they usually start in the choroid. There is a well-known story of a man presenting with a glass eye (due to removal of the eye for malignant melanoma some years previously) and large liver (due to metastases) emphasizing that there may be an interval of years before secondary melanoma develops after excision of the primary site.

Malignant melanomas of the skin are very rare before puberty. Lesions which present many of the features of a rapidly growing melanoma sometimes develop in children and young adults, but these tumours are benign and undergo spontaneous involution. They are referred to as *juvenile melanomas*.

D. Tumours Derived from a Mixture of Tissues

The tumours considered so far all involve one tissue supported by non-neoplastic stroma including blood vessels. Mixed tumours show a variety of neoplastic tissues including both epithelium and connective tissue.

1. Fibroadenoma of Breast

These tumours consist of both neoplastic ductular epithelium and neoplastic stroma. This must be distinguished from epithelial neoplasms, especially scirrhous carcinomas, where there is a considerable stromal support or reaction to the epithelial cells. Fibroadenomas form firm grey nodules which can be shelled out of the surrounding breast tissue. These tumours are benign but occasionally they may become more aggressive to form large lobulated tumours of low grade malignancy called *cystosarcoma phylloïdes* (Brodie's tumour).

2. Mixed Parotid Tumour

These tumours consist of proliferating ductular epithelium in a myxomatous stroma that frequently shows areas resembling hyaline cartilage. It was because of this that these tumours were called 'mixed'. However, there is good evidence to show that the stroma does not consist of true cartilage but rather of pseudocartilage formed by myoepithelial cells proliferating with the ductular epithelium. It will be recalled that small salivary ducts have a double layer of cells, an inner cuboidal or columnar epithelium and an outer myoepithelium. Both types of cells contribute to the neoplasm which is more appropriately called a *pleomorphic salivary adenoma*.

3. Mixed Mesodermal Tumour

Tumours of the endometrium sometimes show neoplastic change involving both the glands and the stroma. The latter may differentiate into a variety of connective tissue components including fibrous tissue, cartilage and striated muscle. These are malignant neoplasms derived from Müllerian duct remnants which may form both mesodermal (endometrial) glands and stroma. The tissues found in these tumours are therefore all derived from one germ layer unlike teratomas described below, which are derived from all three germ layers.

4. Wilms's Tumour or Nephroblastoma

The kidney arises from that part of the primitive mesoderm known as the metanephric ridge. In the kidney therefore, the epithelium and the supporting structures such as smooth muscle fibres and connective tissue all have a common mesodermal origin. Wilms tumour is a malignant neoplasm originating from these primitive mesodermal cells. It usually presents in early childhood and consists of undifferentiated small oval cells with scanty cytoplasm together with differentiated elements including tubules lined by cuboidal or columnar epithelium, primitive glomeruli, fibrous tissue, smooth muscle and even cartilage. The tumour infiltrates neighbouring structures and metastasizes by way of the blood stream to the lungs. Similar embryonal tumours may arise in the liver of infants (*hepatoblastoma*).

5. Teratomas

A teratoma is a true neoplasm composed of multiple tissues of kinds foreign to the part in which it arises. It differs from a hamartoma which is a tumour-like malformation consisting of multiple tissues but of a kind which are all found in the part in which it arises. *Heterotopia* is the term used for tissues which are found in abnormal sites. These may be simply misplaced tissues as, for example, gastric mucosa in Meckel's diverticulum, or they may be neoplastic as in a teratoma.

The most satisfactory explanation of the origin of teratomas is that they arise from pluripotential cells which have for some unknown reason become misplaced during the development of the foetus. The tumours appear to be related to included twins and double monsters by imperceptible gradation. The essential histological feature is that elements of all three germ layers, ectoderm, mesoderm and endoderm, go to make up the tumour, but in a disorderly fashion. Some teratomas behave in an entirely benign fashion, but others are malignant, the malignant tissue ranging in its degree of differentiation. Teratomas are to be observed most frequently in the gonads. Those arising in the ovary are usually benign and cystic and, because squamous epithelium and skin appendages commonly take part in the formation of the cyst wall, they are called dermoid cysts. They tend to become evident during the reproductive period and may reach the size of a grapefruit. The cyst cavity frequently contains putty-like material which consists of flakes of keratin and sebum; hairs commonly project into the cavity. The cyst is mostly thin walled but there is at some point on the circumference a ridge or mound of solid tissue from which bone or teeth may project into the cavity. The substance of the ridge commonly contains skin appendages, respiratory and alimentary epithelium, brain, thyroid, muscle, fibrous tissue, fat and cartilage.

Teratomas which arise in the testis are nearly always malignant. The degree of differentiation varies from mature epithelial and connective tissue elements to anaplastic tumours. An interesting feature in some teratomas is the presence of cell masses strongly resembling chorion-carcinoma of the placenta. These tumours produce chorionic gonadotrophin which gives a strongly positive pregnancy diagnostic test.

Other sites for teratomas are the mediastinum, the sacrococcygeal region and the pineal gland in the brain.

E. The Premalignant State and Carcinoma-in-situ

The concept of premalignancy was first developed by dermatologists to describe skin conditions, not themselves neoplastic, which in some way predispose the affected cells eventually to undergo a frankly malignant change. The concept has since been extended to include similar changes elsewhere in the body. Examples follow.

In the skin, the two best-known diseases are keratosis and leukoplakia. Keratosis consists of a warty lesion which develops in the skin, usually of elderly people who are fair skinned and who have been exposed for long periods to the sun. For the latter reason the lesion is relatively common in Australasia. Histologically the squamous epithelium shows atypical and irregular hyperplastic features which are not so marked as in carcinoma. Leukoplakia is essentially the same pathological change, but is observed in places where moist squamous epithelium exists, such as on the tongue, and vulva. Keratotic lesions produce an excess of keratin, and it is this moistened excess which produces the white plaques indicated by the word leukoplakia. The precipitating factor is still largely unknown; leukoplakia of the tongue was more common in the old days than now, because syphilitic glossitis was an important predisposing lesion.

Other examples of premalignant states are the atrophic gastric mucous membrane of pernicious anaemia in relation to carcinoma of the stomach, hereditary polyposis coli and ulcerative colitis in relation to carcinoma of the large bowel, and chronic inflammation and gall-stone formation in relation to carcinoma of the gall-bladder. In all these cases, carcinoma develops more frequently than can be expected by chance, though the risk varies a great deal from one entity to another. The incidence of carcinoma of the breast is four times as great in association with cystic hyperplasia as in healthy breasts. However, cystic hyperplasia is common and the cancerous risk is considered to be so small that operative treatment is never embarked on in cases of cystic hyperplasia to protect the patient from developing carcinoma. There is no clear dividing line between a premalignant change in epithelium and the entity sometimes diagnosed as 'carcinoma-in-situ'. The latter term implies that the observer considers the involved epithelium, while still confined to its normal situation has histological features indistinguishable from those of frank carcinoma. The term is nowadays most frequently used for changes detected in the cervix uteri, as a result of the contribution of exfoliative cytology to the early diagnosis of malignant disease in this region.

14 The Aetiology of Cancer

It has been shown earlier that cancer consists of proliferation of the cells of a particular tissue in excess of the body's requirements, and of their extension beyond the normal limits of that tissue so that adjacent structures are infiltrated. Cancer cells are thus subject to less restriction of growth than normal ones and are therefore deficient in some of the mechanisms concerned with normal growth. The way in which a normal cell becomes cancerous is still, despite a very great deal of research, unknown, though much information has accumulated about carcinogenic agents and of the conditions under which they produce their effects. This knowledge about cancer has grown both through the study of the disease in human beings and as a result of experimental research on animals. Much more precise information has been acquired in the latter case because inbred strains of animals have been produced which are highly susceptible to one form of cancer or other. Caution has to be exercised in extrapolating conclusions in this field to human disease because animal species differ widely in their reactions to the same stimuli, and because individual human beings, in contrast to the inbred animals, have considerable differences in genetic constitution. Microscopically some cancer cells have been shown to be different from normal ones in the number and arrangement of the chromosomes in the nucleus, but no other fundamental structural differences have yet come to light even under the electron microscope. The altered chromosome pattern could be brought about either through heredity or by way of an environmental factor leading to a mutation in the somatic cell. The knowledge that has been gained about inherited and environmental influences will now be summarized.

Heredity

It has just been pointed out that strains of animals have been bred in which a high incidence of cancer develops; by contrast, there is little evidence that heredity is an important factor in the aetiology of most human tumours. There are a few familial diseases such as xeroderma pigmentosum, neurofibromatosis and polyposis coli in which there is an increased risk of cancer. Family histories of cases of cancer of the breast and of the uterus have been studied from which it has been shown that there has been a significantly higher incidence of cancer in the relatives than the population at large. If one of a pair of identical twins develops cancer, the other is more likely to develop a similar tumour than would be expected by chance.

Environment

Environmental factors which have been shown to exert an influence on the development of cancer are (1) chemical carcinogens, (2) ionizing radiations, (3) physical agents, (4) parasites and (5) hormones.

1. Chemical Carcinogens

The first indication that chemical carcinogens existed came from industry. Scrotal cancer was shown to develop in sweeps, cancer of the skin of hands, arms, and scrotum appeared in workers in shale-oil extraction distilleries and the mule-spinners of cotton mills, and cancer of the bladder is a risk among those working in the rubber and plastics industry and handling aniline dyes. It has also been shown that there is an increased incidence of cancer of lung among heavy cigarette smokers. Experimental verification of the existence of specific chemical carcinogens first came in 1915 when Japanese workers produced cancers in the ears of rabbits which they had painted for many months with tar solutions. Since then a number of other chemical carcinogens have been identified and these fall into three main groups. The first consists of polycyclic aromatic hydrocarbons, which are responsible for the oil, soot, and tar tumours of humans, notably 3–4 benzpyrene. They produce tumours in animals at the site of application or injection. The second group consists of the aromatic amines, which can induce bladder tumours in man. Benzidene and β-naphthylamine are active members of the group. β-naphthylamine also produces similar tumours in dogs, but other species are less susceptible. The amines produce the tumours at a distance from the site of application, and their success depends on their conversion to orthohydroxyamines in the body. The third group of chemical carcinogens are the azo-compounds increasingly used in industry to colour food. Members of the group, the best-known example being 'butter-yellow' (para-dimethylamino-azo-benzene), produce carcinoma of the liver when fed to rats. These therefore are similar to the aromatic amines in that they act at a distance from their site of application.

2. Ionizing Radiations

Skin surfaces, especially of fair-haired people, when exposed for long periods to bright sunlight, are liable to develop keratoses (pre-cancerous lesions) which if untreated sooner or later progress to frank squamous cell carcinoma. In the early years after the discovery of X-rays and radium, workers in the field subjected themselves to undue exposure to these radiations, developed radiation burns as a consequence, and many years later a number suffered from carcinoma of the exposed skin. Excessive unscreened irradiation was also used at one time for treatment of diseases of the thyroid gland and this led subsequently to the development of malignant tumours of the pharynx or larynx. The incidence of such tumours is now negligible because of adequate protective measures. Radium salts if ingested find their way to bones, and may precipitate tumour formation. For example, a number of cases of bone sarcoma occurred among factory girls who had been applying luminous paint containing radium to watch dials for some years previously. They had absorbed the radium by pointing their brushes between their lips. A high incidence of carcinoma especially of bronchus has been shown to exist among the underground workers in the Schneeberg mines in Saxony and the Joachimsthal mines in Czechoslovakia, in both of which the mined ores are radioactive. Carcinoma of the liver has developed in man after intravenous injection of thorotrast (thorium dioxide) used at one time as a contrast medium in radiology. The injected thorotrast was taken up in the reticulo-endothelial (Kupffer) cells in the liver. Carcinoma of thyroid has occurred in some young people whose thymuses had been ill-advisedly irradiated in infancy for the so-called status lymphaticus. Leukaemia has developed with much increased frequency among the Japanese who were exposed to atom bombs at Hiroshima and Nagasaki. The leukaemia arose earlier in those who had relatively the greater exposure. Radiologists have been shown to have a higher incidence of leukaemia than other physicians. There has been an increased incidence of leukaemia among those cases of ankylosing spondylitis submitted to radiotherapy and it is claimed that leukaemia is commoner in children whose mothers have had diagnostic X-ray pelvimetry than in those who have not been so exposed.

In those instances where malignant disease has developed at sites of previous irradiation damage it is reasonable to assume that the radiations were the cause of the cancer. On these occasions when this tissue damage has not been apparent following irradiation, the significance of radiation being carcinogenic in any given situation has been assessed on a statistical basis. In the examples quoted above, the relationship has proved to be highly significant.

3. Physical Agents

Injury often draws attention to the presence of a tumour, as for example a minor fall causing a pathological fracture of bone through a metastatic deposit of carcinoma. However, there is no evidence to show that a single injury can lead to neoplasm. Repeated irritation however, may cause hyperplasia leading to neoplasia. An example of this is seen at the edge of chronic ulcers of the skin, whether due to a sinus draining underlying osteomyelitis (Marjolin's ulcer) gravitational ulcers or lupus vulgaris. Carcinoma sometimes arises in scars of burns or scalds. However, this is an infrequent association suggesting that some other carcinogenic factor may also be operative.

4. Parasites

No *bacteria* have been universally accepted as causes of cancer.

Of the larger *parasites*, schistosomes have been regarded as important causes of cancer of the bladder. These parasites have a very wide distribution in tropical countries, infesting bladder and intestine and causing chronic inflammation and hyperplasia of the mucous membranes. Cancer has been reported to supervene frequently in the bladder, especially in Egypt, but there is doubt at the present time that the cancer is really a complication of schistosome infection, as the latter is practically universal among the Egyptian population and yet carcinoma is relatively uncommon.

Much interest has centred on the possible *virus* origin of cancer. This was first shown to be possible by Rous who in 1911 transferred a sarcoma of the pectoral muscle of a Plymouth Rock fowl to others of the same breed by means of a Berkefeld cell-free filtrate of tumour extract whose potency did not diminish with successive transfers. This demonstration was followed by other successes, also in birds, all the tumours being mesoblastic. In 1922 Shope propagated a fibromatous tumour in wild cottontail rabbits, in the same way as Rous did for his fowls. Later he transferred an epithelial tumour, a squamous cell papilloma, in the same breed of animal by way of Berkefeld filtrates, this papilloma having the ability to spread over the epithelium. It is of interest in this connection, that the common wart of man has been transferred to other individuals by injection of cell free material from the warts, and is thus considered to be of viral origin. Rous found that domestic rabbits were very susceptible to the Shope agent, responding by producing larger, more fleshy, tumours, some of which in the course of time lost their papillomatous character and became invasive in a similar way to human squamous cancer. A proportion of these invasive tumours developed metastases in the regional lymph nodes. Rous later was able to transplant these malignant tumours through several generations of rabbits, though it is of interest that the virus ceased to be extractable when the tumour became malignant. Leukaemia is another variety of malignant disease that can be transferred by cell-free particles both in fowls and in mice. A further example of virus induced tumours in mice which has excited interest lately is the multifocal polyoma. The causative virus was isolated first from a mouse with leukaemia and produces tumours at a number of sites in the body, chiefly in the parotid gland, kidneys, adrenal medulla, breast, thymus, subcutaneous and adipose tissue. Histologically the tumours consist of both benign and malignant epithelial and mesenchymal neoplasms. Both the mouse leukaemia and polyoma viruses have been shown to be widespread in colonies of laboratory mice, but the number of infected animals which develop tumours is relatively low. There is evidence that the vast majority of the mice develop antibodies to the viruses and are thus protected against them.

One of the main difficulties about accepting a virus aetiology for human cancer has been the lack of direct evidence. However, a form of malignant lymphoma, Burkitt lymphoma, has been described in Africa and has a clearly defined geographical distribution, following river valleys and associated with a minimum temperature of 15°C in the coldest season. Such a distribution suggests that a vector, possibly a mosquito, is responsible for its transmission. There is now good evidence to indicate that EB virus may be the cause of the tumour. Recently other virus infections have been found associated with neoplasms, notably nasopharyngeal carcinoma. Care must always be exercised, however, for viruses may be secondary invaders in patients with malignant disease and altered immunity.

The Milk Factor

When the incidence of mammary cancer was studied in the hybrids of high and low cancer strains of mice, it was found that the offspring became most liable to develop cancer if they were born of high cancer strain mothers. Whether the father was of a high or low cancer strain appeared to be of little importance to the offspring's risk, and the tendency to develop cancer followed no recognizable genetic pattern. Bittner found that the operative factor was transferred to the offspring in the mother's milk during lactation. The larger the amount of milk ingested the higher was the subsequent incidence of mammary cancer. This milk factor has been extracted from mammary glands, blood, thymus and spleen of the affected animals, and sometimes also from the cancers themselves. The factor passes readily through the Berkefeld and Seitz filters, is destroyed by heating to 60° C, and survives when frozen and dried; it has also been shown to multiply in the chick embryo. In other words, it has many of the properties of a virus. While this factor has only been isolated for one type of tumour, its discovery is of fundamental importance, as it shows how apparently inherited traits may have in fact other explanations, and also indicates a possible mode of action of a carcinogenic virus.

5. Hormones

The discovery that cholanthrene with its steroid structure was a powerful chemical carcinogen suggested the possibility that spontaneous tumours might sometimes arise from an over-production of endogenous steroids. There is some experimental evidence to support the view that steroids may play a part in the formation of some cancers, but none that they are primarily responsible. It has been found, for example, that if ovaries are removed from mice of high mammary carcinoma strains when they are about six months, the cancer is nearly always prevented. Injections of oestrogens into female mice raise their liability to mammary carcinoma, and prolonged administration also leads to the formation of similar tumours in males. In some strains, interstitial cell tumours of the testis and tumours of the pituitary can also be produced in this way. Since stilboestrol, with its different chemical structure, also produces some of these tumours, it is difficult to accept that the steroid structure of the oestrogens is the factor of carcinogenic importance.

The evidence for the influence of hormones in the production of human cancer is somewhat scanty. Post-menopausal women with cystic glandular hyperplasia of the endometrium, considered to be due to excessive oestrogen production, show an increased tendency to develop endometrial carcinoma. It appears to be possible to halt the progress of prostatic cancer in some individuals either by castration or by the administration of stilboestrol or both. Breast carcinoma seems in some cases to disseminate more slowly if hypophysectomy, adrenalectomy or ovariectomy are undertaken, though no criteria are yet known which will indicate whether such operative procedures will succeed in individual patients.

The Mechanism of Carcinogenesis: the Two-Stage and Protein-Deletion Theories

The Two-Stage Theory

As the result of the accumulated information, briefly touched upon in the preceding pages, it is now widely believed that most cancer cells develop initially from their normal counterparts by way of somatic mutations, and in only a small minority do hereditary influences play their part. The long latent periods between known carcinogenic stimuli and the appearance of the related cancers have led to the view that carcinogenesis may involve a two-stage mechanism. First, normal cells are transformed into latent tumour cells by an 'initiating' agent, then these are converted to freely growing tumour cells under the influence of a second 'promoting' agent. This two-stage mechanism has in fact been shown to operate with some chemical carcinogens in experimental animals. Radiations could well exert their effects by being initiating agents, for only a few over-irradiated individuals develop malignant tumours. It is known that viruses consist of deoxyribonucleic acid (DNA) or ribonucleic acid (RNA) with protective amounts of proteins and lipids. It is possible in the case of virus-induced cancers that these substances get incorporated, with the corresponding elements, in the infected cells altering the genetic make-up of the cells and causing a mutation to cancer. The virus DNA and RNA would in this way act as initiating factors of cancer change. This hypothesis would also explain how viruses often lose their identity when infected cells become cancerous. The Bittner milk-factor could well be another example of an initiating factor, whereas oestrogens and other hormones would appear to be examples of the promoting factor for some tumours, such as those of the breast, uterus, and testis.

The Protein Deletion Theory

Tissues are normally restrained from growing excessively by influences from adjacent structures, the nature of which is still largely speculative, but which are considered to have the activity of antibodies. Some chemical carcinogens are known to become bound to tissue proteins, in which case it might be expected that if cancer cells included such carcinogen-protein complexes their growth would be restrained as a result of the action of antibodies specific for the protein in the complex. If, however, the protein is deleted from such a complex as a result of a mutation, the antibody will no longer be effective against the cancer cell, which would then be able to proliferate and extend into the adjacent tissues in a way impossible for the normal cell.

The two-stage hypothesis is an attempt at an explanation of the way a normal cell becomes cancerous. The protein deletion theory attempts to explain the characteristic behaviour of the cancer cell. Both are speculations but fit the known facts about carcinogenesis better than other hypotheses. They serve therefore as useful guides towards the elaboration of our final understanding of the fundamental problem of the nature and behaviour of the cancer cell.

PART TWO

15 Pathology of the Systems

The number of pages available for the description of the pathology of the systems, or special pathology, are limited, so the account in the following chapters cannot be comprehensive. Students must look to larger reference books for information about the more obscure diseases. The pathology of the illnesses most commonly seen in the wards and the autopsy room will be described here, and space will be given to those rarer entities only when a knowledge of their pathology is contributory to the understanding of general principles.

Table II (p. 134), compiled from the statistics of the Registrar General for England and Wales for 1969, gives some indication of the relative frequency of serious diseases in the various systems.

These are crude figures of the causes of death, being based on information supplied on death certificates. Less than one-third of people come to autopsy when they die so that most of the causes of death given are clinical diagnoses, which inevitably must vary considerably in accuracy. Even when autopsies have been performed, the reasons for the death of the patient are not always clarified. Notwithstanding these objections, some conclusions can be fairly drawn from large numbers, as in these circumstances the inaccuracies of individual diagnoses tend to be ironed out. Further, the statistics compiled from the various countries tend to be largely similar, except for factors due to differences of environment.

There are some observations to be made from Table II. First, the overwhelming importance of diseases of the circulatory system as causes of death should be noted. Including cerebrovascular

TABLE II

Deaths from all causes 1969		579 378
Circulatory system		293 757
Ischaemic heart disease	139 428	
Hypertensive heart disease	10 949	
Chronic rheumatic heart disease	7 512	
All neoplasms		116 035
Trachea, bronchus and lung	29 768	
Large intestine	15 778	
Stomach	12 711	
Breast	10 698	
Lymphatic and haemopoietic system	6905	
Pancreas	4984	
Prostate	4000	
Bladder	3764	
Ovary	3518	
Cervix	2417	
Brain	1740	
Body of uterus	1281	
Respiratory System (excl. neoplasms)		86 156
Bronchopneumonia	34 747	
Chronic bronchitis	29 881	
Cerebrovascular disease		79 728
Accidents, poisons, violence		23 300
Motor vehicle traffic accidents	6558	
Diseases of infancy		14 391
Perinatal mortality	6639	
Digestive system (excl. neoplasms)		14 105
Genito-urinary system (excl. neoplasms)		8071
Endocrine, metabolic, nutritional diseases		6652
Diabetes mellitus	4720	
Congenital malformations		4472
Suicide		4326
Infective and parasitic diseases		3922
Tuberculosis	1840	
Blood and blood forming organs (excl. neoplasms)		1878

disease they account for 373 485 deaths or approximately two-thirds of the total. This situation arises because a frequent cause of death in this group is what might be called degenerative cardiovascular disease, a feature linked with the process of ageing. The number of deaths due to this cause is increasing because, as a result of the considerable advances in clinical medicine, people are living longer now than their predecessors did. This is shown, for example, by the low position in the table occupied by death from infective diseases, a total of 3922, which is to be compared with the 20 000 deaths from this cause twenty years ago. Much of this reduction is due to the improved treatment of tuberculosis, deaths from this cause falling from 16 000 in 1950 to less than 2000 in 1969. These figures for infective diseases do not include those of respiratory origin such as influenza, bronchitis and pneumonia which do much to swell the figure for respiratory deaths and which have also steadily declined over recent years because of antibiotic therapy. The importance of neoplasms as a cause of death is to be noted, these diseases being responsible for 20 per cent of the total, and coming second to those due to circulatory disorders.

Outstanding in importance amongst neoplasms are those arising in the bronchus and lung. This is particularly so in men, but is by no means negligible in women in whom it accounts for about half as many deaths as carcinoma of the breast, approximately the same number as carcinoma of the stomach and twice as many as carcinoma of the cervix. In 1969 more than 24 500 deaths in men alone were due to carcinoma of the bronchus and lung. This compares with a total of 6500 deaths for all persons from road traffic accidents. One of the most impressive and alarming changes in the pattern of disease has been the increase in lung cancer in the past twenty years. In 1949, the death rate from lung cancer for males was approximately 350 per million male population. In 1969 it had risen to more than 1000 per million and for the age group 65–74 it was nearly 6000 per million. Much of this increase can be attributed to cigarette smoking. Many of the 30 000 deaths from chronic bronchitis are also associated with this habit. It will be found helpful to refer back to the common causes of death in dealing with the various systems to appreciate their relative importance in clinical practice.

16 The Circulatory System

Atheroma

This is an extremely common disorder affecting the arterial tree, being increasingly more probable the older the patient, but not directly linked with the phenomenon of ageing, as it may be absent in some old people and very extensive in some who are relatively young. Not only is atheroma common, but it is pre-eminent among diseases liable to cause the death of the sufferer, and, as is the case with many of the other lethal diseases, the ultimate cause is still unknown.

Macroscopic Picture

The lesions of atheroma may be divided into three categories of fatty streak, plaque and complicated lesions. Superficial yellow fatty streaks are common in the intima of the aorta in children and young adults. There is an uncertain relation between these streaks and atheromatous plaques which give rise to clinical disease. Atheromatous plaques increase in severity and prevalence particularly after the age of 35 years in men and 55 years in women. With more severe disease, complications develop with calcification or haemorrhage in the plaque, surface thrombosis and ulceration.

The atheromatous plaque is a focal swelling involving the intima of the aorta and its main branches, the coronary arteries and the cerebral arteries. The abdominal aorta immediately above the bifurcation is the part most liable to be involved, though plaques surrounding the orifices of the small branches leading off it are often early features. The uncomplicated plaque is yellow or cream coloured, firm with a smooth endothelial surface. When calcified it forms a hard plaque or it may appear brown if there has been haemorrhage into it or thrombosis on its surface; more severe lesions may ulcerate. The fatty material has the consistency of putty when not calcified. Cross section of coronary arteries show that the plaques form a crescent resulting in a narrowed and eccentric lumen. The media is not directly affected, but it may become thin beneath the thicker intimal plaques due to pressure and impairment of oxygen diffusing from the lumen through the thickened intima. This leads to fibrous replacement of the muscle and results in an aneurysm, a phenomenon most frequently seen at the distal end of the aorta.

Microscopic Picture

The superficial fatty streaks show accumulation of fat droplets, and later foamy macrophages, in the sub-endothelial connective tissue. The established plaque shows eccentric proliferation of loose intimal fibro-elastic tissue, rich in mucopolysaccharides and containing thin walled capillaries. In the deeper layers of the intima, cholesterol and its esters are deposited appearing in sections as clear sharp-pointed clefts having been dissolved out in the preparation of the tissue. In the same area there is frequently evidence of extravasation of blood in the form of fibrin and free red cells or, where the latter have been broken down, in the form of brown granules of haemosiderin within histiocytes. Where fat and haemorrhage are present, calcification is common. Ulceration of the intimal surface causes thrombosis and subsequent organization. The underlying media is thinner due to partial fibrous replacement of the elastica and muscle. Aneurysm formation is associated with loss of muscle from the media, and deposition on the inner aspect of laminated organizing thrombus and on the outer by fibrous tissue with chronic inflammatory cells in the adjacent connective tissues.

Complications

The complications of atheroma mainly arise from the reduction of blood supply to the part supplied. This blood supply may become gradually reduced because the increasing amount of atheromatous change slowly narrows the lumen of the artery, or it may become suddenly shut off through the formation of an obliterative thrombus or an embolus, from the ulcerated atheromatous surface, impacting farther down the arterial tree. A gradual reduction of blood supply leads to replacement fibrosis in the part supplied, a sudden cut-off to infarction. These complications make their clinical impact mainly in three situations: (a) the heart, (b) the brain and (c) the legs. Aneurysm formation is a less common cause of symptoms (d).

(a) *The Heart: Myocardial Fibrosis and Infarction*

Atheroma is common in the coronary arteries, and much more so in the left artery than the right. The former is most frequently affected in its main section and in its anterior descending branch; the left circumflex branch is somewhat less commonly involved. Progressive narrowing of the arteries leads to the clinical syndrome of angina pectoris. This form of pain arises because the cardiac muscle is ischaemic, as a result of which it will show replacement fibrosis. Grey streaks may therefore be visible in the affected myocardium, and microscopically strands of fibrous tissue will be seen to run between the atrophic myocardial fibres. Occlusive thrombosis is a relatively common event in the coronary arteries, and is a frequent cause of death. The effect on the heart will depend on the site of the occlusion, and the extent of atheroma in the coronary artery system. Healthy coronary arteries act more or less as end-arteries, but the more narrowed they become as a result of atheroma, the more their terminal branches tend to anastomose with each other. In most instances, when occlusive thrombosis occurs, there is evidence of widespread atheroma throughout the coronary arteries. Coronary artery occlusion (or coronary thrombosis) leads to myocardial infarction. The infarction may lead to immediate cardiac failure, and indeed this is a common cause of sudden death. Under these circumstances no change will be visible in the myocardium. If the patient survives the thrombosis and dies a little later, the affected myocardium will show the changes of infarction, the picture depending on the time interval between the thrombosis and the death of the patient. The most common site of the infarct is in the anterior two-thirds of the left ventricle and interventricular system, particularly in the region of the apex, since this is the area supplied by the anterior descending branch of the left coronary artery. Infarcts are much more likely to develop in the left ventricle than the right, and are practically unknown in the auricles. A recent infarct reveals itself as a yellowish brown area in the myocardium, surrounded by a hyperaemic zone. A healed infarct will consist of a fibrous scar. If the infarct reaches the pericardium, this will become inflamed and covered with a fibrinous exudate (fibrinous pericarditis) leading eventually to fibrous adhesions between the visceral and parietal pericardium. The endocardium is usually spared because oxygen diffuses from the ventricle, but if it is involved it will excite the deposition of mural thrombi within the recesses of the muscular trabeculae.

There are complications of myocardial infarction other than death from acute cardiac failure. The infarction may be superimposed on an already fibrotic myocardium, so that chronic cardiac failure may ensue. The endocardial thrombi may break off into the circulation, and the resulting emboli may lead to the formation of infarcts in other organs, the most important of which, clinically, is the brain. The infarcted myocardium is softened in the earlier stages and if large enough may rupture leading to the formation of a haemopericardium with resultant death from cardiac tamponade. Alternatively the rupture may involve the interventricular septum causing a ventricular septal defect, or it may result in rupture of a papillary muscle and sudden mitral incompetence. The fibrous scar of a healed infarct may so thin the myocardial wall that aneurysmal dilatation occurs with subsequent risk of rupture. This is most likely to take place at the apex where the myocardium is normally thinner than elsewhere. Other complications of myocardial ischaemia include cardiac arythmias. Atrial fibrillation may result in the formation of thrombi in the atrial appendage with the risk of emboli from this site. An infarct may involve the conducting system resulting in heart block.

(b) *The Brain: Cerebral Thrombosis and Embolism*

Cerebral infarction is a relatively common lesion in adults and is usually due to atheroma. It may follow occlusion of a branch of one of the cerebral arteries, most commonly the middle cerebral. However, it may also follow occlusion of the internal carotid artery just beyond its origin from the common carotid artery in the neck. Many cerebral infarcts follow embolism of a cerebral artery by a fragment of thrombus or atheromatous debris from one of these larger more proximal arteries.

(c) *The Legs: Intermittent Claudication and Infarction*

The gradual narrowing of the main arteries in the legs as a result of atheroma leads to the symptoms of intermittent claudication, or muscular pain in the calves on exercise. No pathological changes can be identified in the limb except for the severe atheroma. Occlusion of a proximal segment of the arterial supply to the legs does not usually produce any further symptoms because blood usually passes through collateral arteries. Occlusion of one of the more distal branches may result in infarction of the part of the foot supplied.

(d) *Aneurysm Formation*

This relatively uncommon complication of atheroma has already been mentioned (p. 137). It occurs most frequently at the distal end of the aorta, and may reach the size of a hen's egg. The aneurysm may either leak blood slowly or may rupture producing more acute abdominal symptoms.

Aetiology of Atheroma

In spite of the widespread nature of the disease and the seriousness of its complications, the aetiology of atheroma is still largely obscure. Several factors appear to be linked with the development of atheroma. *Age:* The disease increases in frequency with age, but the correlation is not absolute, for it may be minimal in old age and severe in the young. *Sex:* Men are more frequently affected than women, although the incidence increases rapidly in women after the menopause. *Hypertension:* Atheroma is more frequent in association with hypertension and this applies particularly in the pulmonary circulation, but there is not a close relationship, for atheroma may be severe in normotensive individuals or absent in those with severe hypertension. *Mechanical stress:* Atheromatous plaques tend to be localized and most severe at the bifurcation of large arteries or at the ostia of small branches where turbulence is greatest. *Blood lipids:* The lipid content of the aorta increases with age. The lipids which accumulate in the intima and in atheromatous plaques are quantitatively similar to blood lipids. Lipids are normally carried in the blood conjugated to protein to form lipoproteins. Most of the lipoprotein can be divided into two classes: (1) low molecular weight, high density, α lipoproteins and (2) high molecular weight, low density β lipoproteins. Patients with atheroma tend to have high blood levels of β lipoproteins, fasting triglycerides and cholesterol. They also have high cholesterol: phospholipid and lipid: protein ratios. Diseases such as diabetes mellitus and myxoedema which are associated with a high blood cholesterol also show an increased incidence of atheroma. Administration of thyroxine to myxoedematous patients lowers the level of blood cholesterol and of β lipoproteins. Diets containing largely unsaturated (vegetable and fish) fats are associated with lower levels of blood cholesterol than diets containing much saturated (butter, eggs, meat) fat. The high incidence of atheroma in the western hemisphere may partly be accounted for by the high concentration of animal fat in the diet.

There are two principal theories of the development of atheroma. The *imbibition or filtration theory* relates atheroma to blood lipid, particularly to the level of β lipoprotein. This theory postulates that relatively insoluble lipid passes into the vessel wall from the lumen. Because of the absence of blood and lymph capillaries from the intima, the lipid accumulates in the deep intima. However, this theory requires additional factors to explain the localization of atheromatous lesions within vessels. It is postulated that local mechanical factors, such as turbulence of blood, cause the localization of the lesions and this can be demonstrated experimentally. Once fat is deposited in the intima it induces the fibrous reaction forming part of the atheromatous plaque.

The *incrustation or thrombogenic theory* suggests that atheroma is due to thrombi being deposited on the vessel wall. Initially these consist of platelets and fibrin. The foam cells of the early lesion represent histiocytes which have phagocytosed platelets rich in lipoprotein. When mural thrombi have formed they become covered by endothelium, the blood breaks down to give the cholesterol and blood pigment, while organization of the thrombus gives rise to the fibrous tissue. This theory explains the irregular distribution of atheroma in the body and the eccentric lesion in the vessel. It is probable that both these theories are involved in the production of the established lesion.

The incidence of atheroma does not appear to have altered much in the past fifty years, but the incidence of coronary thrombosis has greatly increased. This suggests that other factors, increasing the tendency to thrombosis, may be important in the genesis of coronary occlusion. In this connection it is noteworthy that some lipids are augmentors of blood coagulation, and that platelets have been shown to be more sticky than normal in this disease.

Hypertension

Definition

Hypertension means a raised blood pressure. There is still no general agreement for a blood pressure figure which represents the upper limit of normal, partly because it may fluctuate under emotional and other stresses, partly because it increases with age, and partly because its measurement is commonly not wholly objective. The diastolic pressure reading is considered to be more important than the systolic, and a persistent level of over 100 should be regarded with suspicion.

Aetiology

Hypertension most commonly exists without any coexistent disease when it is known as *essential hypertension.* The most significant aetiological factor is renal disease and for this the term ***renal hypertension*** is used. The commoner renal diseases involved are proliferative glomerulonephritis and pyelonephritis. Experimentally hypertension is most easily produced by creating renal ischaemia by clamping a renal artery. The counterpart in human disease of renal artery stenosis is rare. Other renal diseases which give rise to hypertension include polycystic kidneys, and amyloidosis. There are many endocrine causes of hypertension. A tumour of the adrenal medulla, phaeochromocytoma, which is capable of secreting noradrenaline and adrenaline excessively may give at first intermittent hypertension, followed by sustained hypertension. Although uncommon, this is important diagnosis for surgery offers cure if undertaken before irreversible renal damage has been caused by the hypertension. Tumours of the adrenal cortex, leading either to excess production of glucocorticoids and Cushing's syndrome, or to the excessive production of aldosterone and Conn's syndrome, may also cause hypertension. Sometimes the cause is due to hyperplasia of the adrenal cortex rather than neoplasm. Hydatidiform mole and chorion carcinoma of the placenta associated with excess production of chorionic gonadotrophin may also cause hypertension. Another important cause of hypertension is toxaemia of pregnancy, but the precise mechanism is uncertain. Finally congenital malformations such as coarctation of the aorta may give rise to hypertension proximal to the obstruction.

In most of these cases the disease persists for several years and in many instances it is silent until an advanced stage. It is referred to as *benign hypertension* but this is a misnomer as it frequently is the cause of death. *Malignant hypertension* is diagnosed if a patient suffers from a rapidly increasing blood pressure, which is associated with the presence of papilloedema.

Pathology

The blood pressure is the product of cardiac output and peripheral resistance. In hypertension from all causes, the important factor is increased peripheral resistance. In the early stages of the disease, no structural changes can be identified, so that the diagnosis remains clinical. This finding also indicates that the first change is a functional narrowing of the smaller blood vessels. When structural changes appear, the first elements to become altered, as might be expected, are the distal components of the arterial tree, the arterioles. The walls of these vessels become thickened and the lumens narrowed. The thickening is partly due to hypertrophy of muscle, and partly to increase of fibrous tissue. Characteristically a glassy eosinophilic change supervenes—*hyaline arteriolosclerosis*. This change can take place throughout the body, but, perhaps significantly, it only has a high correlation with the development of hypertension when observed in the kidney. By contrast, similar changes in the arterioles of the Malpighian corpuscles of the spleen are common, and are of no hypertensive significance. The development in other viscera is of intermediate significance.

The primary arteriolar sclerosis in the *kidney* causes two further changes. First, because of the increased peripheral resistance, the arteries undergo hypertrophy in an attempt to compensate for it. The thickening of the artery walls can be appreciated macroscopically, because the cut surfaces tend to be much more prominent than normal. Microscopically three elements of the artery contribute to its increase of size. The muscle coat hypertrophies, there is a concentric new formation of fibrous tissue in the intima, and the internal elastic lamina reduplicates, or splits into two or more layers. Secondly, because of the narrowed arteriolar lumens, the blood supply becomes reduced to the tissues distally. An arteriole supplies a small number of nephrons, and these will undergo replacement fibrosis when the arteriole is sclerotic. Not all arterioles are affected equally, so that small foci of fibrous tissue are interspersed between normal surviving nephrons, which may in fact show compensatory hyperplasia. The result of these changes is the production of the characteristic finely granular capsular surface of the kidney, slight loss of detail in the cut surface, and moderate reduction in the overall size of the kidney. The kidney of essential hypertension is thus one of the causes of contracted granular kidney. The arcuate and larger arteries will be more prominent than normal when the cut surface of the kidney is examined.

In order to maintain an adequate blood flow in the face of increasing peripheral resistance, the left ventricle of *the heart* eventually undergoes hypertrophy which may in time become very striking (cor bovinum). The left ventricular cavity usually remains relatively small unless cardiac failure supervenes.

Malignant hypertension, like essential hypertension, can exist without demonstrable arterial lesions. There are two changes which are diagnostic of this state. First, the renal arterioles and intraglomerular capillaries may show fibrinoid change. This is similar histologically to hyaline arteriolosclerosis but tends to be a deeper pink, and is, in fact, due to necrosis of the vessel wall with deposition of fibrin or fibrinogen in the wall. The second vascular lesion is a very loose lamellated ('onion-skin') fibrous thickening of the arterial wall. Where the arteriolar walls are necrotic, small haemorrhages are liable to develop, and when the blood supply is reduced rather rapidly to the distal tissues, small infarcts may arise. The vascular lesions of malignant hypertension may be seen in other situations in the body beside the kidney.

Complications

The majority of people with essential hypertension eventually suffer from, and die of *heart failure*. A common episode is acute left ventricular failure, the development of a sudden crisis of dyspnoea because the failure precipitates pulmonary oedema. Frequently, however, the failure is more gradual, the strain being taken up by both ventricles so that ultimately congestive cardiac failure develops. *Apoplexy or cerebral haemorrhage* is the next most common complication of essential hypertension. This is most frequently seen in the region of the internal capsule and may be of considerable extent. Such a haemorrhage may be accompanied by other small haemorrhages elsewhere in the brain. *Chronic renal failure* is less common than the other two complications in essential hypertension, but, in malignant hypertension, death is most frequently by way of uraemia. In addition to the effects of hypertension, there is often severe atherosclerosis which further complicates the cardiac, cerebral and renal disease.

Mechanism

Much of the experimental work on renal hypertension indicates that renal ischaemia plays an important role. Clamping of one renal artery results in hypertension, but if the clamp is removed before vascular changes have developed in the opposite kidney, the hypertension resolves. However, if release of the clamp is delayed, the hypertension is irreversible. It has been shown that an inactive pressor substance, renin, is produced by the juxtaglomerular cells of the afferent arterioles as they enter glomerular tufts in the renal cortex. Renin acts on a circulating globulin, angiotensinogen, to produce an active pressor substance, angiotensin. This has a direct effect on blood vessels causing vasoconstriction and leading to hypertension. It also stimulates the production of aldosterone by the adrenal cortex and this aldosterone leads to sodium and water retention contributing to the hypertension. However, if both kidneys are removed and the animal kept alive by repeated dialysis, hypertension still develops (renoprival hypertension) and this is assumed to be due to an extrarenal pressor substance called vasoexcitor material (VEM) which is normally inactivated by the kidney.

Other factors may also play an important part, particularly neurogenic factors. Elevation of the blood pressure can be shown to follow emotional stimulation. Sympathectomy is effective in reducing the blood pressure in a number of patients. It may well be that in essential hypertension, emotional stimulation causes the initial hypertension, and the resulting arterial disease causes renal damage which perpetuates the hypertension.

Rheumatic Heart Disease

Rheumatic heart disease, an illness of temperate climes, appears to be less common than it used to be. *The acute attack* (acute rheumatism) is a delayed inflammatory reaction following an infection by *Streptococcus pyogenes* (p. 94). It affects the heart, the joints and the nervous system. In the heart all layers are involved. The endocardium is the seat of a chronic inflammatory reaction mainly in the region of the valves, though the posterior wall of the left auricle is often also implicated. The naked-eye evidence of inflammation is the presence of small wart-like vegetations, composed largely of platelet clumps and fibrin. On the valves, these lie along the line of closure. The valves on the left side of the heart are much more commonly affected than those on the right, and the mitral valve more frequently than the aortic. More than one valve can be affected in an individual patient. No naked eye change can be identified in the myocardium, though it is here that the characteristic Aschoff nodes occur. These are found in the loose perivascular connective tissue of the myocardium and consist of fibrinoid necrosis surrounded by histiocytic mesenchymal cells (Anitschkow myocytes), lymphocytes and giant cells. As the lesion heals it leaves a fibrous scar. Fibrinous pericarditis may develop and results in an adherent pericardium. Joints are commonly involved but rarely give permanent disability. There are focal areas of mucoid or fibrinoid change in the synovium, and sometimes lesions resembling Aschoff nodes. In the subcutaneous tissues especially around joints, rheumatic nodules may form. These are similar to nodules found in rheumatoid arthritis and consist of fibrinoid necrosis surrounded by palisaded histiocytes and lymphocytes. The lungs may show interstitial pneumonitis and there may be lymphocytic perivascular cuffing of vessels in the brain associated with chorea. Acute rheumatism of the heart may heal, but this recovery carries with it an increased risk of subsequent attacks compared with normal people. Some cases will die of acute cardiac failure; on the other hand acute rheumatism may develop over the years into chronic rheumatic heart disease. The latter may also appear out of the blue in an individual who cannot recollect having had rheumatic fever.

Chronic rheumatic heart disease is dominated by a progressive sclerosis of valvular endocardium. The mitral valve is most frequently affected. The valve cusps thicken and fuse, and the chordae tendineae shorten, thicken, become paler and sometimes matted. Mitral stenosis thus develops with a rigid orifice, and there may be in addition calcification of the valve leaflets. Such stenotic valves are inevitably also incompetent, but the disease occasionally leads predominantly to a dilatation of the valve in which case the effects of incompetence are more striking.

The aortic valve is also frequently affected in chronic rheumatic heart disease. The aortic valve cusps adhere at their contiguous edges, and when the sclerotic cusps shrink towards their points of attachment, incompetence results. The valve becomes stenosed rather than incompetent when the tendency of the cusps to adhere dominates over their tendency to retract. Super-added calcification sometimes complicates the stenosis.

Lesions are much less common in the valves of the right side of the heart, the tricuspid valve when affected being liable to incompetence, and the pulmonary artery to stenosis.

The diseased valves throw a strain on the heart and changes develop, particularly in the pulmonary circulation, which lead eventually to congestive cardiac failure. The obstruction to flow through the mitral valve causes dilatation of the left atrium and hypertrophy of the atrial muscle. When atrial fibrillation supervenes, thrombus is very liable to form in the atrial appendage. Back pressure on the pulmonary circulation causes congestion of the lungs and the escape of red blood cells into the alveoli. The haemoglobin is broken down to haemosiderin where it may be seen in macrophages—'heart-failure cells'. The chronic congestion stimulates fibrous proliferation in the alveolar walls, and this thickening, together with the haemosiderin pigmentation, gives rise to the macroscopic appearance of 'brown induration' of the lungs. When pulmonary hypertension is severe, atheroma develops in the pulmonary artery and the right ventricle hypertrophies. Right ventricular failure follows with systemic venous congestion. Disease of the aortic valve results in dilatation and hypertrophy of the left ventricle, and when this fails pulmonary oedema develops. Other important complications of chronic rheumatic heart disease are thrombotic emboli arising from the left atrial appendage and passing into the systemic circulation, and subacute bacterial endocarditis. Subacute bacterial endocarditis will be described below.

Bacterial Endocarditis

This name is given to bacterial infection of the heart valves, which exists in two distinctive groups, acute and subacute. *Acute bacterial endocarditis*, which is rare, is a terminal event in a severe acute septicaemic infection, originating elsewhere in the body and caused usually by *Streptococcus pyogenes*, pneumococcus or *Staphylococcus aureus*. The infection may affect either healthy or previously diseased valves. The vegetations are larger and more crumbly than in acute rheumatism, tending to ulcerate the affected cusps and chordae tendinae and to erode into the underlying myocardium. They consist of platelets and fibrin but include clumps of bacteria, and inflammatory cells. The friable vegetations are very liable to break off to form emboli which lead to the formation of infected infarcts which tend to suppurate. Untreated, the patients do not survive long, more because of the septicaemia than the endocarditis.

Subacute bacterial endocarditis is different from the acute form in the pathogenicity of the infecting organisms. The disease has an insidious onset, and, when untreated, a protracted course. The patient may present as a pyrexia of unknown origin (PUO) which may be accompanied by symptoms due to embolic phenomena. The disease is usually due to infection with *Streptococcus viridans*, a relatively avirulent organism, in the vast majority of cases. This gets into the blood stream transiently in normal people from the region of the teeth during mastication, but is more liable to do so if dental caries is present. In affected patients the organisms settle in the valves because they are diseased, the two principal abnormalities being chronic rheumatic heart disease and, in the case of the aorta, congenitally bicuspid valves. The orifice of a patent ductus arteriosus may also be infected. Because of the decreased incidence of chronic rheumatic heart disease and of improved dental hygiene, the disease is not so common as it used to be. Its previous gloomy prognosis has been ameliorated by the advent of antibiotic therapy. The vegetations are large and crumbly like the acute ones, but are often more extensive because of the longer course of the disease. The microscopic structure of the vegetations is similar to that in the acute form, except that they show the features of organization at the point of attachment to the valve. Extension to the left auricular endocardium may occur as in rheumatic heart disease. Erosion and ulceration of the valve cusps are less common complications than in acute bacterial endocarditis, embolization tending to dominate the scene. The brain, spleen, kidney and skin are common sites for the emboli, which, in contrast to those of the acute disease, do not suppurate. This is because the organism is less virulent, and also antibodies have been able to develop to high titre.

In addition to emboli which occlude medium-sized arteries, some patients develop proliferative glomerulonephritis due to the deposition of immune complexes of antigen and antibody in the glomerular capillary wall. When the untreated patient dies it is usually because of exhaustion after a long infective illness, sometimes because of the cerebral embolic complications, and less commonly because of cardiac failure.

Other Forms of Endocarditis

Verrucous Endocarditis or *Libman-Sacks* endocarditis is due to systemic lupus erythematosus. Small vegetations occur on the mitral and tricuspid valves and less frequently on the semilunar valves. The vegetations may occur anywhere on the cusps, but they differ from those of rheumatic fever in that they may extend on to the undersurface of the cusp. The valves show mucoid change and foci of fibrinoid necrosis, later leading to fibroblastic proliferation.

Nonbacterial, Thrombotic Endocarditis is found in patients dying after protracted debilitating diseases such as advanced malignancy. The vegetations are found particularly on the mitral and aortic valves and consist largely of fibrin and platelets. They are thought to occur as an agonal event.

Endocardial Fibroelastosis is found particularly in children and results in considerable thickening of the endocardium, most commonly on the left side of the heart. There is accompanying hypertrophy of the myocardium. Anoxia appears to play an important part in the development of the lesion and many cases are associated with congenital anomalies. A similar subendocardial fibrosis occurs in East African adults following necrosis of muscle fibres. It appears to be due to a metabolic or nutritional defect.

Carcinoid syndrome due to excessive secretion of 5-hydroxytryptamine usually by metastatic carcinoid tumour arising in the ileum, gives rise to widespread fibrous thickening of the endocardium in the right side of the heart. This fibrosis results in pulmonary stenosis.

Other Lesions of the Heart

Myocarditis

Sudden death may occasionally be due to myocarditis. It may be possible to identify the infecting organisms and these include (1) pyogenic bacteria in cases of septicaemia, (2) diphtheria, where the damage is due to the exotoxin of the bacteria producing fatty degeneration of the cardiac muscle, (3) viruses especially those of poliomyelitis, measles and mumps and (4) parasites such as toxoplasmosis and trypanosomiasis (Chagas's disease). The infecting organism may not be known, examples being sarcoidosis and acute interstitial myocarditis (Fiedler's myocarditis).

Pericarditis

The fibrinous pericarditis of acute rheumatism and myocardial infarction have already been mentioned. Bacterial pericarditis may complicate acute inflammatory conditions of the lungs. Pericarditis is also a terminal complication of uraemia. It is a feature of malignant tumour infiltration, usually from the lung.

Chronic pericarditis is a feature of tuberculosis and can also arise without known aetiology (chronic constrictive pericarditis). Macroscopically the changes of acute or chronic inflammation will be seen, with an exudate forming in the cavity, being serofibrinous or fibrinopurulent in the acute cases and predominantly serous in the tuberculous or malignant cases, the latter often being bloodstained. Small pericardial effusions are common events in the post-mortem room. They are transudates, usually due to the causes of generalized oedema, e.g. cardiac failure.

Tumours

Primary tumours of the heart are very rare. 'Rhabdomyomas' of the cardiac muscle are hamartomas sometimes found in patients with tuberose sclerosis. Atrial myxomas arise in the vicinity of the interatrial septum, more commonly on the left. They are usually polypoid tumours and may block the mitral orifice when the patient is erect. Secondary tumours, especially those arising in the lung, commonly infiltrate the pericardium and myocardium.

Congenital Heart Disease

This is an important cause of perinatal mortality, and minor grades are compatible with adult life. Only the more common disorders are mentioned. *Fallot's tetralogy* consists of a subvalvular pulmonary stenosis with a ventricular septal defect, an overriding aorta and right ventricular hypertrophy. As deoxygenated blood from the right ventricle enters the aorta, there is cyanosis of varying degree. *Eisenmenger's complex* is similar, without pulmonary stenosis. *Patent foramen ovale:* as a valvular defect this is a common finding at post mortem. When there are large *atrial or ventricular septal defects* the shunt of blood is usually from left to right. *Patent ductus arteriosus:* the ductus is normally obliterated by eight weeks of extra-uterine life, but when patent it allows a shunt of blood from the aorta to the pulmonary artery. *Coarctation of the aorta* most commonly occurs between the origin of the left subclavian artery and the ductus arteriosus, but occasionally occurs in other situations. It may be associated with a bicuspid aortic valve. The complications of congenital heart disease include cardiac failure, pulmonary hypertension, cyanosis, hypertrophic pulmonary osteoarthropathy and subacute bacterial endocarditis.

Syphilitic Aortitis

This has become much less common of recent years largely because of the response of syphilis to therapy with penicillin. The first part of the aorta above the level of the diaphragm is most commonly affected. The aorta appears dilated and thin. The intima is usually the seat of extensive atheroma, but between the fibrous plaques it is characteristically wrinkled. Histologically there is intense cuffing of the vasa vasorum of the aorta by chronic inflammatory cells, particularly plasma cells. The lumina of these small vessels tend to be obliterated by reactive thickening of the walls, so that the blood supply, and hence the nutrition of the aortic media is impaired. As a consequence, there is degeneration of the elastic and muscle fibres with replacement of the media by vascular scar tissue.

Syphilitic aortitis which proceeds only to minor dilatation of the vessel does not lead to the development of symptoms. These will arise only if the aortic valve ring is involved or if an aneurysm develops in the aorta. The valve ring is in fact commonly affected, and its dilatation leads to incompetence of the valve. This change can be inferred to have occurred if the commissures between the valve leaflets are seen to be wider than normal. The leaflets themselves may become somewhat fibrotic. The aortic incompetence means that some of the blood expelled into the aorta during systole regurgitates into the left ventricle during diastole at a time when it is receiving blood from the lungs by way of the left auricle. The left ventricle enlarges partly because it becomes more dilated to accommodate the increased amount of blood during diastole, and partly because it hypertrophies in order to expel the greater load in systole. Left ventricular failure is thus a common end-result in this disease. If the destruction of the elastic coat of the aorta by syphilis is sufficiently severe at any point, a saccular aneurysm develops. The aneurysm, as it grows, is liable to erode neighbouring structures such as the lung, mediastinum, oesophagus, vertebral column or pleura, producing a wide range of symptoms. Sooner or later the thinned fibrous wall may rupture, leading to a sudden massive and fatal haemorrhage. Microscopically the wall of the aneurysm will consist of an outer layer of fibrous tissue and an inner layer of organizing laminated thrombus. Chronic inflammatory cells are usually present in the adventitia.

Other Arterial Lesions

Endarteritis obliterans is a commonly observed change consisting of concentric fibrous thickening of the arterial intima. The change is seen in those situations where the artery is not required to supply such an abundant blood supply as in the past. Examples are in the post-partum myometrium, in the floor of a chronic peptic ulcer, and in the wall of a chronically inflamed gall-bladder. In the last two instances the metabolic activities of the new formed fibrous tissue are less than the epithelium and smooth muscle it has replaced. This phenomenon protects the sufferer from peptic ulcer from having as many massive haemorrhages as he might otherwise have on the occasions when arteries become eroded in the ulcerating process.

Polyarteritis Nodosa. The arteries resemble those in the Arthus phenomenon (p. 89). The disease may develop without any obvious precipitating factor or it may appear as a hypersensitivity reaction to drugs or infections. Some patients present with an illness similar to rheumatoid arthritis and progress to polyarteritis nodosa. Adult males are affected more commonly than women. The lesions are found most frequently in medium-sized muscular or small arteries in the kidneys, skeletal muscle, heart, liver and gastro-intestinal tract. The skin, central nervous system and joints are also commonly involved. In the kidneys, as well as arteritic lesions, there may be involvement of capillaries in the glomerular tuft. Renal failure and hypertension are important complications of this disease. Some patients respond to corticosteroid therapy but many die as a result of renal, cardiac or cerebral damage.

Temporal Arteritis. This is a focal inflammatory reaction involving the temporal arteries usually of old people, leading to intractable headache. Other arteries may be less frequently affected, one of the more common being that to the eye, leading to blindness. Microscopically there is active chronic inflammation of the arterial wall and fibrosis of the intima. Granulomatous foci consisting initially of polymorphs but later of lymphocytes, plasma cells and foreign-body giant cells which develop in relation to the degenerate internal elastic lamina. The disease may extend to involve other sites including the kidney.

Wegener's Granulomatosis. This disease has many features similar to those of polyarteritis nodosa. However, it characteristically involves the respiratory tract with granulomatous arteritis in the nasopharynx and lungs. There is usually renal involvement and other organs may also be affected. Classical polyarteritis nodosa does not commonly involve the lungs.

Thromboangiitis Obliterans (*Buerger's Disease*). Besides atheroma, thromboangiitis is another cause of intermittent claudication, occurring in younger people than the former. At the time of symptoms, the artery shows occlusion by a recanalized thrombus, which is considered to be the end-result of inflammation of the vessel wall, though no persisting inflammatory reaction can usually be identified. The disease has only rarely been observed in the acute stage. In the chronic stage of the disease the veins may also be affected and the perivascular fibrosis spreads to include the adjacent nerves. Many consider that thromboangiitis is not an entity but represents the results of atherosclerosis, thrombosis or embolism, alone or in combination.

Other Aneurysms. The so-called *dissecting aneurysm* of the aorta consists of a splitting of the media by blood driven in from the lumen through a breach in the intima. The blood may track back into the pericardium leading to cardiac tamponade or forward down the aorta eventually re-entering the iliac branches or escaping through the adventitia to produce torrential bleeding. The dissection arises because of cystic accumulation of mucopolysaccharides in the media (cystic medial necrosis) which weakens the wall. This may result from a congenital abnormality of collagen (Marfan's syndrome) or follow hypertension. It may also be associated with coarctation of the aorta. *Congenital or 'berry' aneurysms* may develop at the junctions of the main arteries in and around the circle of Willis at the base of the brain, as a result of congenital structural defects in the arterial walls. Rupture of such an aneurysm is the basis for subarachnoid haemorrhage. They may also be associated with hypertension and polycystic kidneys. *Mycotic* aneurysms are usually small and arise as a result of bacterial infection of the arterial wall often as a complication of bacterial endocarditis.

Veins

The superficial veins of the legs of older people are liable, through valvular incompetence, to become dilated and tortuous. Such *varicose veins*, which are very common, show replacement of the muscle by fibrous tissue. Thrombi sometimes form in them, but they more usually produce symptoms through the production of eczema or even ulceration of the overlying and undernourished skin.

Thrombi develop very commonly in the deeper veins of the leg, and are associated with the complication of pulmonary emboli (see pp. 42, 44). Thrombi may form in bacteria-infected veins, but this is a much less frequent clinical problem. *Thrombophlebitis migrans* is a disease which may complicate carcinoma, particularly of the pancreas. The vein is occluded by thrombus and the wall infiltrated by inflammatory cells.

Lymphatics

Acute lymphangitis is best known in the form of the thin red line which may be seen in the skin adjacent to an acutely infected focus. *Local obstruction of lymphatics* produces lymphoedema of the part normally drained. The most likely clinical examples are when the vessels are obliterated by malignant disease (e.g. the peau d'orange in carcinoma of the breast), after radiotherapy (e.g. lymphoedema of the arm following irradiation of the breast and axilla for carcinoma), or as a result of congenital absence of lymphatics (Milroy's disease). In the tropics, infestation of the lymphatics by a filarial parasite is very liable to produce lymphoedema, especially of the legs and scrotum (elephantiasis). The chronic lymphoedema so produced gives rise to elephantiasis of the affected part.

Tumours of Blood Vessels

Angiomas, arising either from blood or lymph capillaries are common in the skin. They may consist either of capillary vessels or of larger blood spaces—cavernous haemangiomas which give the 'port wine stain'. The latter when occurring on the head may be associated with similar dilated vascular spaces in the underlying bone, meninges and brain. Cavernous lymphangiomas in the neck are called cystic hygromas.

Glomus tumours occur mainly in the skin of the hands. They are small but very painful and microscopically can be seen to consist of capillaries surrounded by uniform sheets of glomus cells which normally are found surrounding the endothelium in specialized structures referred to as glomus organs.

Angiosarcomas are rare. Those arising from blood vessels can be divided into tumours of endothelial origin and those of pericyte origin. The latter sometimes resemble smooth muscle tumours, e.g. uterine 'fibroids'. Lymphangiosarcomas are found following chronic lymphatic obstruction. Angiosarcomas are highly malignant tumours, freely metastasizing as may be assumed from their close relationship with the lumina of vessels.

Kaposi's sarcoma is usually classified with angiosarcomas but the cell of origin is uncertain. It occurs in parts of Central Europe and Africa most commonly in adult males. Multiple tumours in the skin and viscera consist of small blood vessels and spindle cells which appear sarcomatous.

17 The Respiratory System

The Lungs

It is in the post-mortem room rather than the operating theatre that pathological abnormalities in the lungs are most commonly observed. Before discussing individual diseases, certain changes will first be described which may arise from more than one cause. The normal lung is spongy and dry when cut. In the infant and the country dweller it is mottled pinkish grey in colour, whereas that of the adult town-dweller is greyish black, because of the considerable amount of soot which the lung accumulates from the atmosphere.

Congestion

The acutely congested lung is dark purplish red, and when cut and compressed will exude more blood than normal. Common causes of acute congestion are left ventricular failure and acute inflammation. The lung of chronic venous congestion due to mitral stenosis tends to be tougher than normal, and the cut surface presents a lighter chocolate brown colour. Microscopically the alveolar capillaries of congested lungs are conspicuous because they are filled with blood. In chronic congestion there are in addition an abundance of histiocytes containing haemosiderin in the alveolar lumina ('heart failure cells').

Oedema

Pulmonary oedema makes the lung more solid than normal macroscopically, and on palpation transmits the sensation given by a wet sponge. The cut surface exudes abundant clear fluid on compression. Microscopically the alveolar lumina are filled with a clear lightly eosinophilic exudate. Common causes are acute left ventricular failure, early acute infection, and conditions producing generalized oedema such as renal disease. Occasionally it will be produced as an occupational hazard as a result of the inhalation of a chemical irritant or following cerebral injury.

Fibrosis

Fibrosis of the lung can result from a wide range of precipitating factors. Infective causes are unresolved pneumonias, tuberculosis, chronic bronchitis and bronchiectasis. It may result from malignant disease, sarcoidosis and excessive radiotherapy. It is a dominant feature in the occupational hazard of pneumoconiosis when it follows inhalation of irritant dusts such as silica and asbestos (silicosis, asbestosis). It may occur focally or be diffusely distributed, and the naked-eye picture is one of firm pale grey plaques or streaks.

Collapse

Collapse of lung occurs when the air normally contained in the alveoli becomes absorbed and is not replaced through respiration. As might be expected, the volume of the collapsed lung is less than normal so that the pleural surface becomes wrinkled. The lung is more solid than normal and of uniform deep purple grey (or 'slaty') colour. Collapse arises as a result of obstruction of the bronchial tree supplying the area, the commonest cause of the obstruction being undrained bronchial secretion, but others are neoplasms and inhaled foreign bodies. It will also result through compression by an expanded pleural cavity as in effusion or pneumothorax. Massive collapse is the name given to the acute emergency liable to arise after abdominal operations, but which is precipitated by the common cause, undrained bronchial secretions.

Atelectasis

This is the state of a lung when it has never been expanded by air, and is therefore a phenomenon of stillbirth or the neonatal period. Birth injuries to the brain are considered to play an important part in its production: aspirated amniotic fluid may be contributory. As might be expected, the general appearance is that of collapse.

Hyaline Membrane Disease

Although hyaline membranes may be found lining respiratory bronchioles, alveolar ducts and alveoli at all ages, it is in the newborn that it is of greatest importance. Premature infants, those born by Caesarian section and of mothers with diabetes mellitus are particularly prone to develop respiratory distress and hypoxia some hours or days after birth. These infants often die, and the collapsed lung is airless. Section reveals eosinophilic hyaline membrane lining the distal air passages. It is believed to be due to a deficiency of surfactant. This substance lowers the surface tension of the alveoli in normal lungs and allows them to expand.

Pneumonia

Definition

Pneumonia can be defined as the filling of the air spaces of the lung with inflammatory exudate. The exudate may involve the whole or part of a lobe. In the former instance it is termed lobar pneumonia. If the consolidated alveoli are clustered round the terminal portions of the bronchial tree, the inflammation is termed bronchopneumonia.

Aetiology

Pneumonia can be a primary inflammation of the lung substance or it can be secondary to another disease process such as carcinoma or chronic bronchitis. The infecting organism is frequently undetermined, for many cases recover and the bacteriological findings in the sputum do not necessarily reflect the microbial state in the pneumonic lung. Recent careful laboratory studies on cases of pneumonia illustrate these points. Viruses were isolated from a quarter of radiologically diagnosed pneumonias from patients over 15 years and from a seventh in those younger than 15. The viruses were most commonly the influenza and para-influenza viruses and adenoviruses. When samples of sputum from patients with pneumonia were cultured, nearly half failed to grow any organisms which might be regarded as being possibly pathogenic. Pneumococci were grown from a third of the samples, *Haemophilus influenzae* from one fifth, and staphylococci much less frequently. The tubercle bacillus can at times produce pneumonic consolidation, but this is now a rare manifestation of the disease.

Pathology

Lobar pneumonia is not now commonly seen in the post-mortem room. It virtually never follows the old-fashioned dramatic clinical picture, but tends to be the somewhat surprising finding in an old person, who may well have been afebrile and, perhaps, discovered unconscious at his or her home. Macroscopically four stages are recognized. The first is one of *congestion* and is followed by an exudative phase in which the lung is red and solid (*red hepatization*). In the third stage the lung is paler grey and drier (*grey hepatization*). In the patient who recovers, the lung returns to its normal state (*resolution*). Microscopically, in the first stage there is congestion of the alveolar capillaries and this is followed by exudation of red cells, fibrin and neutrophil polymorphs into the alveoli. In the stage of grey hepatization the alveolar capillaries are collapsed and bloodless, the exudate now consisting mainly of neutrophil polymorphs. During resolution the alveolar exudate liquefies, and part is coughed up and part absorbed.

Complications of Lobar Pneumonia

The inflammatory reaction usually spreads to the pleural surface so that pleurisy occurs. This may cause a pleural effusion which is rich in protein and fibrin and has the characteristics of an exudate. There may be a purulent exudate giving an empyema. Infection may spread to give pericarditis. The lung parenchyma may break down to form a lung abscess. This is commoner with some types of pneumococci and staphylococci. Instead of resolution of the pneumonic exudate, this may become organized to form a carnified or fibrotic lung.

Bronchopneumonia is a much commoner picture in the post-mortem room. Macroscopically the involved lung appears congested and oedematous, and on palpation may feel lumpy. When the cut surface is examined, the diagnostic feature is a cluster of minute pale solid nodules surrounding small bronchi or bronchioles. Histologically, the bronchiolar wall is inflamed and its lumen filled with polymorphs; the adjacent alveoli show similar changes. The more peripheral alveoli are congested and oedematous, the inflammatory reaction here being at an earlier stage of evolution. With severe infections, adjacent solid areas coalesce to produce an incomplete lobar pattern. Bronchopneumonia is more serious than lobar pneumonia, for it always causes some destruction of the lung parenchyma. In old people already suffering from chronic lung disease, this additional destruction further reduces the pulmonary reserve.

Suppurative bronchopneumonia, in which multiple abscesses form in the consolidated areas, is a common picture in staphylococcal infection, a disease of considerable gravity.

The commonest picture of pneumonia seen at the present time consists of the non-specific combination of congestion and oedema; this is because of the antibiotic therapy which is practically invariably given. The disease which used to be referred to as primary atypical virus pneumonia is now recognized as being caused by a mycoplasma and not a virus. It is frequently associated with the presence of cold agglutinins in the blood and may be suspected histologically if the exudate in the alveolar wall consists predominantly of histiocytes and lymphocytes rather than polymorphs.

Influenza. This infection is a common winter illness but every few years it occurs as a pandemic. Certain strains of the virus are more pathogenic than others and cause serious disease with a high mortality particularly in the elderly and very young. At post-mortem the lungs are congested and oedematous with areas of haemorrhage. The trachea and major bronchi show violaceous congestion and contain thin haemorrhagic secretion. Microscopically there is mononuclear cell infiltration of the alveolar septa and walls of the larger air passages. The alveolar lumen may contain haemorrhagic oedema but polymorphs are usually scanty unless there is a secondary bacterial infection giving bronchopneumonia.

Lipid pneumonia is either exogenous or endogenous. Exogenous lipid pneumonia is caused by the inhalation of lipid, the two common sources being cod liver oil and oily nasal drops. Endogenous lipid pneumonia may be found distal to a bronchial obstruction and the lipid comes from the lipoprotein in cell membranes being broken down and ingested by histiocytes.

Chronic Bronchitis and Emphysema

These two diseases are considered together because they are so commonly associated, and are the basis of a considerable morbidity among the older section of the population in this country. Epidemiological studies have shown that the combination is commoner in our climate than in a tropical one, in town than in the country, among the old than the young, and among the poor than the rich.

The clinical yardstick for *chronic bronchitis* is the production of an excessive amount of sputum. The constant pathological change is an increased thickness of the glands of the bronchi with a preponderance of mucus secreting cells. The opening of the ducts of the glands on to the surface of the bronchi also become abnormally wide. The bronchial walls are infiltrated by inflammatory cells during acute episodes of infection, but do not usually become further damaged. Chronic bronchitis produces progressive ill health because it helps in the development of emphysema in the lung alveoli connected with the inflamed bronchi.

Emphysema may be defined as the lung condition in which there is an increase beyond the normal in the size of the air spaces distal to the terminal bronchiole, either from dilatation or destruction of their walls. The classification of emphysema depends mainly on the distribution of dilated air spaces within the secondary lung lobule. *Centrilobular emphysema* shows dilatation or destruction of air spaces around the bronchiole, whereas *panacinar* (*panlobular*) emphysema shows this change throughout the lobule. A rare variety of emphysema is confined to the paraseptal region of the lobule. Adjacent to scars, the emphysema is unrelated to the lobule and is related only to the scarring—*focal emphysema.*

Centrilobular emphysema is frequently found in association with chronic bronchitis. It is suggested that the recurrent attacks of bronchiolitis damage the wall of the bronchiole and adjacent alveoli, causing scarring around the bronchiole with subsequent compensatory dilatation of the neighbouring respiratory bronchioles and alveoli. This dilatation results in an increase in the dead space of the lung and a decreased area for exchange of gases. Pulmonary hypertension develops with right ventricular hypertrophy leading to cor pulmonale. The pulmonary arteries become atheromatous. The cause of this pulmonary hypertension is not clear. It is due in part to spasm of the small arteries as they cross the dilated air spaces in the centre of the lobule and in part to opening up of anastomoses between the pulmonary arteries and bronchial arteries which contain blood at systemic blood pressure. Destruction of lung tissue also increases the resistance of the pulmonary vascular bed. Eventually the heart fails and chronic venous congestion develops. These patients are referred to as 'blue bloaters' because of the cyanosis and oedema of cardiac failure.

Panacinar emphysema is less frequently associated with chronic bronchitis, and although the amount of lung damage may appear greater, pulmonary hypertension is less noticeable. However, as their total area for gas exchange is reduced they are dyspnoeic. Increased respiratory effort maintains reasonable oxygen tensions in the blood. They are therefore not cyanosed and are called 'pink puffers'.

Macroscopically emphysema may be inconspicuous unless the lung is fixed inflated. Sometimes, the emphysema develops into polypoid projections near the surface, called bullae. These are liable to perforate, leading to escape of air into the pleural cavity—pneumothorax.

Pneumoconiosis

This is a group of lung diseases caused by the inhalation of dust usually as an industrial hazard.

Silicosis is due to the inhalation of silica dust most commonly in coalmines, or quarries where stone containing silica has to be cut. The larger particles are removed by the action of cilia in the major air passages, but the particles of less than $3 \mu m$ enter the alveoli where they are ingested by macrophages. These macrophages enter lymphatics which they block and cause a fibrous reaction. Surrounding this there is focal emphysema. These patients also have a high incidence of tuberculosis which may contribute to the lung scarring.

Anthracosis. Carbon does not itself cause fibrosis, but in mines the carbon of coal often contains small quantities of silica. The carbon inhaled by city dwellers appears to be inert in the lung.

Asbestosis is caused by the inhalation of asbestos (magnesium silicate) in the manufacture of material or in industries concerned with pipe lagging and brake lining. It is an important cause of pulmonary fibrosis, and also causes an increased incidence of carcinoma of the lung and mesothelioma of the pleura.

Farmer's lung is an allergic form of dust disease caused by the inhalation of a thermophilic actinomycetes in hay (see page 89). It leads to pulmonary fibrosis. Other allergic dust diseases include *byssinosis* (cotton dust) and *bagassosis* (sugar cane).

Bronchiectasis

Bronchiectasis is a condition in which the bronchi become dilated either in cylindrical or saccular form. The disease is most common in the lower lobe bronchi and is associated with the production of abundant foul sputum, which cannot be drained away as effectively as in the normal. Microscopically the wall of the dilated bronchus is usually heavily infiltrated with chronic inflammatory cells and the muscular coat appears thinned. There is destruction of cartilage and metaplasia of the lining epithelium to a stratified squamous pattern. Ulceration of the mucous membrane will take place in the later stages, and there will be a varying degree of collapse and fibrosis of the surrounding lung. Bronchiectasis is considered to be due to (1) weakening of the supporting tissue of the bronchial wall by inflammation, (2) contraction of the surrounding fibrous tissue, and (3) increased pull by inspiration as a result of the collapse of the surrounding lung. It is usually a sequel to severe acute infections, such as measles and whooping cough in the earlier years, though it is possible that a congenital abnormal thinness of the bronchial tree is a contributory factor in some cases. There is often associated nasal sinusitis and the drainage of the infected secretion into the lungs during sleep may cause other cases. The disease is becoming less common nowadays probably as a result of the more effective treatment by antibiotics. Lung abscesses, metastatic abscesses, especially in the brain, and amyloid disease are well-recognized complications.

Tuberculosis

Pulmonary tuberculosis, for years a major infective illness cutting down the young in their prime, has become so much less frequent of recent years that many sanatoriums have ceased to be used for its treatment. This is a result of the discovery of specific antibiotic therapy grafted on to a rise in the general standard of living and hence nutrition. The disease is now liable to present in atypical fashion; for example it may be discovered to be the cause of respiratory infection in old people.

The primary infection leads to the development of a 'Ghon focus', which is usually midzonal and subpleural in situation. It consists of the characteristic granulomatous inflammatory reaction which may become caseous; the hilar lymph nodes draining the focus may also become infected. The Ghon focus heals to form a fibrous or calcified nodule in the vast majority of cases. With re-infection, the classical post-primary lesion develops at the apex of one or both lungs, consisting at first of a localized pneumonic consolidation before the characteristic tubercles develop. This again heals in the great majority of people, often without symptoms, to produce the sometimes calcified apical scars so commonly seen in the lungs of people in civilized communities. In some individuals, however, the disease will spread and become clinically evident. The caseation in individual tubercles coalesces and the softened lung tissue may be removed by expectoration so that a cavity develops. The lung in the untreated case becomes increasingly disorganized and fibrosed with continued spread of the infection, usually by way of the lymphatics. The state of fibrocaseous tuberculosis eventually results, which is very much more difficult to cure, and which in fact may lead to death of the patient through progressive deterioration of respiratory reserve. The pleura may become involved in the chronic progression of the disease with the result that fibrous adhesions develop, or sometimes bronchopleural fistula forms, leading to pneumothorax and tuberculous empyema. The progression of the disease may become more active as a result of rupture of infected material into a bronchus and spread therefrom into the related alveoli, leading to pneumonia which in its most active form is lobar in distribution (caseous pneumonia or 'galloping consumption').

Another common presentation of respiratory tuberculosis in the early post-primary phase is the pleural effusion. The fluid is clear and may be abundant, containing many lymphocytes from which tubercle bacilli can frequently be cultured. The effusion usually subsides completely even without specific therapy, leaving no radiological evidence of underlying pulmonary infection. Biopsy and endoscopy studies have shown, however, that the affected pleura contains a number of tubercles. The amount of effusion and the rapidity with which it forms suggests that the fluid exudes from much of the pleural surface, probably as a manifestation of the hypersensitive state.

The common complication of pulmonary tuberculosis is spread of the infection to elsewhere in the body. A primary focus, particularly that in a hilar lymph node, is liable to erode into a blood vessel, and the flooding of tubercle bacilli into organs, particularly when resistance is low, leads to the formation of *miliary tuberculosis.* This serious event was an important cause of death in children in pre-antibiotic days because of the development of tuberculous meningitis. Tubercle bacilli draining into the thoracic duct may give rise to miliary tuberculosis in the lungs. Spread from a tuberculous cavity via the major air passages may involve the intestinal tract as a result of swallowed sputum, leading to tuberculous ulcers of the bowel, ileocaecal 'hyperplastic' tuberculosis or fistula-in-ano. Renal tuberculosis is a blood-borne infection, usually starting from an active pulmonary lesion. Amyloidosis is a complication liable to develop in cases of long standing pulmonary tuberculosis. The pulmonary fibrosis associated particularly with the secondary infection is liable to cause focal emphysema and bronchiectasis. Carcinomas sometimes arise in old tuberculous scars following metaplasia of alveolar epithelium at the periphery of the scar.

Sarcoidosis

The lesion of a sarcoid reaction is similar to a tubercle except that caseation does not occur and acid fast bacilli cannot be demonstrated. The majority of cases of sarcoidosis show diffuse pulmonary infiltration which may scar to give a 'honeycomb lung'. Lymph nodes, spleen, liver, skin, uveal tract, salivary and lacrimal glands are all commonly involved. There may be bone lesions in the hands similar to those of hyperparathyroidism and this may be accompanied by a raised serum calcium and nephrocalcinosis. A few cases eventually show features of tuberculosis, but in the majority the aetiology remains obscure. In addition to the characteristic histological changes, the diagnosis may be confirmed by a positive *Kveim test.* This test depends on the intradermal injection of a phenolized extract of a sarcoid lymph node with the development of a characteristic sarcoid reaction six weeks later. A local sarcoid reaction is sometimes seen in lymph nodes draining malignant lesions, or in the lungs, skin and lymph nodes in berylliosis, but these cases do not have a positive Kveim test and they should not be diagnosed as sarcoidosis.

Carcinoma of Bronchus

Bronchial carcinoma is a disease of considerable importance because it is now the commonest fatal cancer, and in this country in men aged 45–64 deaths from lung cancer are now equal to deaths from all other forms of cancer together. It enters into the differential diagnosis of most of the persistent respiratory ailments, and of a good many others presenting outside this system. Careful epidemiological studies have shown that the way is open to diminish, and perhaps largely obliterate, its incidence. These investigations have shown beyond any reasonable doubt that the incidence of this cancer parallels the incidence of cigarette smoking, and that the risk is greatest among the heaviest smokers. Cigarette smoke contains both cancer initiators and cancer promoters (p. 129). The former include polycystic aromatic hydrocarbons and the latter phenols, fatty acid esters and free fatty acids. Laboratory animals have developed lung cancer after being trained to inhale cigarette smoke. In man the risk of developing lung cancer is increased approximately 30 fold for those smoking 30 cigarettes per day.

Macroscopic Appearance

The macroscopic picture of carcinoma of the bronchus varies extremely widely as any regular visitor to the post-mortem room knows, and thus it practically defies description. The tumour may start anywhere in the bronchial tree and in any lobe. It is commoner in the larger primary divisions of the bronchi than elsewhere. The tumour may be so small that meticulous dissection by an experienced pathologist is necessary to reveal it, on the other hand it may be so extensive as to involve much of the lung, spreading even to cover the whole of the pleural surface. The frequency of pleural involvement is indicated by the frequency of pleural effusion as a presenting symptom, from which malignant cells may be identified in a cytological specimen. The tumour may consist merely of a roughening of the bronchial surface, which can be associated with a considerable infiltration of the surrounding lung tissue, or it may cause occlusion of the bronchial lumen, either by growing into it as a polypoid tumour, or by cicatrizing it by growing round in the wall. The less common periphrally situated tumours often appear as spherical masses, with which no communication with a bronchus can be clearly demonstrated. Some of these arise in a fibrous scar in the lung, e.g. at the site of healed tuberculosis. These scars frequently contain atypically disposed air cells lined by cuboidal epithelium which are believed to be the starting point of such tumours. On section the tumour most commonly presents a pale grey or brown cut surface. A wide variety of secondary changes can occur in the lung drained by the affected bronchus. It can be congested, oedematous, consolidated, emphysematous, collapsed or bronchiectatic, and more than one feature can be present at the same time. The tumour may cavitate as a result of necrosis so that fluid levels may be seen radiologically.

Microscopic Picture

This can vary almost as much as the macroscopic picture, though there are three broad subdivisions of epithelial structure: (a) squamous cell carcinoma, (b) oat cell carcinoma, and (c) adenocarcinoma, the frequency descending in the above order. Squamous cell carcinoma occurs particularly in the major bronchi near the hilum of the lung. It is the principal form of carcinoma associated with cigarette smoking and is much commoner in men.

Oat cell carcinoma was formerly referred to as undifferentiated carcinoma, but it has distinctive features with small, oval hyperchromatic nuclei which distinguish it from other undifferentiated carcinomas of squamous or glandular origin. Recent evidence indicates that it may be derived from Kultschitzky cells in the bronchial mucosa forming part of the argentaffin system better known in the alimentary tract. Adenocarcinoma is relatively more frequent in women and occurs in the second or third order of bronchi about midway between the hilum and the pleura. Rarely carcinomas may arise from alveolar lining cells and spread through the alveoli. These tumours cannot be distinguished by biopsy from metastatic adenocarcinoma in lung spreading in a similar fashion.

Spread

The different patterns of spread are legion. A minute tumour may be associated with many and widespread metastases. A large tumour infiltrating locally may show few or no secondary growths. The direct spread is commonly into the hilum and on into the mediastinum with the result that the great vessels may become encased or compressed, the recurrent laryngeal nerve infiltrated, and the pericardium widely permeated. A tumour arising near the apex of the lung may give the superior pulmonary sulcus syndrome (Pancoast's syndrome). This consists of pressure on the brachial plexus giving pain and wasting of the arm, and pressure on the cervical sympathetic chain giving Horner's syndrome. Lymph node metastases are common and may be distant, though those at the hilum, in the neck, and axilla, are most commonly involved. The hilar node enlargement may be considerable and produce mediastinal obstructive symptoms. As the lung is a vascular structure in immediate communication with the systemic circulation, it is not surprising that blood-borne metastases are common and may be widespread. Cutaneous metastases, for example, are often the first diagnostic sign that the tumour exists in a patient. Cerebral metastases are the commonest malignant tumours in that tissue. Bronchial carcinoma is one of the likely primary sites to produce osteolytic skeletal metastases. The liver is very frequently infiltrated, and the tumour appears to have a predilection to metastasize to the adrenal glands.

Systemic Manifestations

Besides producing sometimes unexpected symptoms and signs by way of metastases, bronchial carcinoma can also be responsible for other syndromes for which the presence of tumour cannot be directly implicated. Endrocrinological syndromes are particularly associated with oat cell carcinoma. These include (1) Cushing's syndrome with hyperplasia of the adrenal cortex, (2) inappropriate secretion of antidiuretic hormone leading to hyponatraemia which cannot be attributed to bone metastases. Neurological syndromes include a peripheral neuromyopathy and cerebellar degeneration. Other syndromes include dermatomyositis, hypertrophic pulmonary osteoarthropathy and thrombophlebitis migrans.

Bronchial Adenoma

These tumours occur earlier in life and there is not the same discrepancy in sex incidence as there is in bronchial carcinomas. They appear in the larger bronchi as polypoid growths, but the great bulk of the tumour is locally infiltrative in the bronchial wall. Histologically, two patterns are found, carcinoid tumours and cylindromas. The former resemble the carcinoid tumour of the alimentary tract and a few produce the carcinoid syndrome (flushing, cyanosis, diarrhoea and occasionally pulmonary stenosis) with an increased urinary excretion of 5-hydroxyindoleacetic acid (5–

HIAA). Cylindromas resemble salivary gland tumours. Both types occasionally metastasize.

Pulmonary Hamartoma

These tumour-like malformations are usually detected on routine chest X-ray where they are seen as rounded shadows in the lung field. They consist of abundant bronchial cartilage intimately mixed with glandular epithelium—hence their alternative name of adenochondroma. They are benign.

The Larynx and Trachea

Acute infection of the larynx frequently occurs as part of an upper respiratory infection. The development of the inflammatory reaction may so interfere with the normal function of the vocal cord that hoarseness results. An important acute infection is diphtheria, characterized by the development of a pseudomembrane consisting of necrotic debris, exudate and fragments of shed epithelium. The exotoxin produced by the organism produces systemic effects on the heart and nervous system. *Tuberculous ulceration* may develop secondarily to spreading pulmonary infection. *Oedema*, from any cause involving the larynx, may produce acute respiratory distress necessitating a tracheotomy (e.g. angioneurotic oedema). Oedematous fibro-epithelial *polyps* are common lesions on the vocal cords ('singer's nodes'); they are brought about by constriction of lax mucous membrane by the movements of the cords during talking and singing. Recurrent squamous cell *papillomas* may at times be seen and are probably viral in origin.

Squamous cell carcinomas may develop in the larynx accounting for rather less than 1 per cent of all malignant tumours in the body. The tumours may be intrinsic, occurring either just below, on, or just above the vocal cords, or extrinsic, arising on the epiglottis, aryepiglottic folds or pyriform fossa. They spread by local invasion or lymph node metastases; blood stream spread is uncommon. The extrinsic tumours spread more readily and therefore have the worse prognosis.

Serious pathological conditions are uncommon in the trachea. It takes part frequently in the inflammation produced by upper respiratory infections; malignant disease is distinctly rare.

Further Reading

Royal College of Physicians Report (1971) *Smoking and Health Now*. London, Pitman.
Spencer, H. (1968) *Pathology of the Lung*. 2nd edn. Oxford, Pergamon.

18 The Tissues of Head and Neck

The Lips

Squamous cell carcinoma of the lip accounts for 1 per cent of all malignant tumours. It is frequently preceded by non-syphilitic leukoplakia. It is commoner in the older age groups and much more frequent in men than women. There is an increased incidence among pipe smokers and fair-skinned individuals exposed to excessive sun. The tumour occurs particularly on the lower lip, infiltrates locally and ulcerates. Metastases are usually to the submandibular or pre-auricular lymph nodes. The ulcerated tumour is liable to become severely infected.

The Tongue

Atrophy of the glossal epithelium with flattening of papillae together with desquamation of the mucocutaneous junction at the angle of the lips (angular stomatitis) occurs in deficiency states of which lack of iron and vitamin B_{12} are important examples. Iron deficiency produces atrophy at the sides first and the tongue is un-inflamed, compared with the total atrophy and inflammatory reaction of vitamin B_{12} deficiency. Intestinal disorders leading to riboflavine and nicotinamide deficiencies, and oral antibiotic therapy, produce similar lesions.

Squamous cell carcinoma of the tongue makes up 1 per cent of all malignant tumours. The incidence is approximately equal between the sexes, and the tumour is commoner among the older age groups. Leukoplakia, which is nowadays rarely due to syphilis, is a significant pre-existing lesion for the carcinoma developing in the anterior part of the tongue. The tumour spreads in the same way as carcinoma of the lip and shows the same liability to infection.

The Mouth

Mucous retention cysts are common, consisting usually of small swellings in the buccal cavity, arising as a result of blockage of the duct of one of the many salivary glands that open into the mouth.

Teeth frequently become carious, and the tooth sockets may be the seat of chronic, sometimes purulent, inflammation, producing apical abscesses, gumboils and pyorrhoea. Infected tooth sockets are believed to be the portal of entry for *Actinomyces israeli.* This organism, causing actinomycosis, sets up an acute inflammatory reaction in the jaw which extends to the overlying skin. The tissue becomes wood-hard and multiple skin sinuses discharge the characteristic 'sulphur granules'. Staining of the buccal mucosa adjacent to teeth is seen in chronic poisoning with heavy metals, e.g. lead. Pigmentation of the oral mucosa may be racial, or genetic, as in the oral pigmentation and intestinal polyposis of Peutz-Jeghers syndrome. Addison's disease may also cause buccal pigmentation.

Dentigerous cysts are squamous epithelial lined cysts around unerupted teeth, whereas *dental cysts* are squamous epithelial lined cysts around root abscesses. Sometimes the inflammation produces a local swelling of the gum, an *epulis*, which consists largely of the reactive fibrosis to the inflammation.

Infections of the mouth may be viral, bacterial or fungal. Herpes simplex is a common recurring oral viral infection. Vincent's gingivitis produces acute necrotizing inflammation caused by *Borrelia vincentii* and fusiform bacillus. Monilial infection (thrush) is a common complication of oral antibiotic therapy; it also occurs in children and debilitated adults. Small white spots contain the mycelial network. The infection may spread into the air passages and oesophagus. The exanthemata show oral lesions, Koplik's spots of measles being well known. Lesions are also seen in the mouth in chickenpox and smallpox.

Adamantinoma is a tumour arising from the enamel organ of the developing tooth. The majority occur in the lower jaw and present as expansile, locally infiltrative tumours. The histological pattern resembles the enamel organ and consists of a reticulum of stellate cells surrounded by columnar or cubical cells. Another tumour which presents as swelling of the jaw is the *Central African lymphoma* of children (p. 127). *The gums* become diffusely swollen following anti-epileptic drugs and in some cases of leukaemia; *ulcers* may appear in the buccal cavity and throat in leukaemia, and through agranulocytosis. Small painful, often recurrent, sometimes multiple, ulcers are common in the mouth; called *aphthous ulcers*, their aetiology is still obscure. *Squamous cell carcinoma* apart from that of the tongue occurs most commonly in the floor of the mouth. Salivary tumours may be seen, especially in the palate, a reminder that numerous small glands exist within the buccal cavity.

The Throat

Acute inflammation, with ulceration and deeper extension (quinsy), occurs in the tonsil and at the back of the throat and is usually due to *Streptococcus pyogenes*. Diphtheria is nowadays rare. *Chronic inflammation* of the tonsil leads to considerable lymphoid hyperplasia particularly in the young.

Squamous cell carcinoma is the commonest malignant tumour of tonsil and pharynx; in the latter situation it tends to be poorly differentiated and of relatively poor prognosis. Anaplastic carcinomas in this area are sometimes referred to as *lymphoepitheliomas*. Often being small, they may be overlooked and present first with lymph node metastases in the neck. Because of the abundant lymphoid tissue in this region, *malignant lymphoma* is only a little less frequent than carcinoma. The natural history is that of malignant lymphoma in general.

The Nose and Nasal Sinuses

This area differs from the mouth and throat in that, being part of the respiratory system, it is lined by ciliated stratified columnar epithelium. Hypersecretion is therefore as prominent a feature of *infection* as it is in the bronchi. This will be obvious to most through experience of that common virus infection, the cold. The mucous membrane also becomes congested, and it is the combination of congestion, hypersecretion, and slowing of ciliary action which is responsible for the stuffiness so typical of the disease. In the later stages, the voluminous watery secretion gives way to one which is more scanty, viscid, and purulent, due in part to secondary bacterial infection.

The continued production of secretion and its ineffective drainage through their orifices are responsible for the unpleasantly painful symptoms of acute and chronic *sinusitis*, and treatment, both medical and surgical, is directed towards improving the drainage. Chronic infection causes lymphoid swelling to occur at the back of the nose in the young, producing the well-known obstructive syndrome of *adenoids*.

Inflammatory changes also result from *hay fever* or allergic rhinitis, and eosinophils are prominent in the inflammatory exudate. A moderately common late result of both types of inflammation or a combination of them is the development of *nasal polyps*, which tend to be recurrent. They consist of oedematous and inflamed submucosa covered by normal epithelium. Nasal papillomata differ from polyps in that they are covered by transitional epithelium, tend to recur and eventually to give rise to invasive tumours. *Nose bleeds* are common phenoma, which are usually of trivial importance, but which on occasions may be so persistent and recurrent that serious anaemia develops. Most arise through congestion following virus infection, some follow trauma, others occur in hypertensives and patients with blood diseases. A few arise through vascular abnormalities (telangiectases).

Carcinoma is the commonest malignant disease here as elsewhere in the oronasopharynx. It is commoner in Chinese and also has a higher incidence in workers in wood and nickel industries. The cell type of the carcinoma varies; some are squamous, some are straightforward adenocarcinomas, and others are salivary tumours. Lymphoepitheliomas occur here as in the tonsil. Malignant lymphomas are not rare. Malignant tumours here tend to have a relatively poor prognosis, because of the inaccessibility for complete surgical excision. An unpleasant progressive granulomatous and ulcerating inflammatory lesion of unknown aetiology occasionally develops in this region, the so-called *malignant granuloma*. It appears to be closely related to polyarteritis nodosa. Pulmonary and renal vascular lesions occasionally complicate the pharyngeal granuloma and are then referred to as Wegener's granuloma.

The Ear

The *pinna* undergoes the same pathological changes as the skin generally. The *external auditory meatus* is relatively free of common pathological lesions apart from superficial infections. The *ear-drum* may perforate after the exudates from secondarily infected virus inflammations, such as the common cold, extend to and accumulate in the middle ear causing distension of the drum. If the infection does not subside quickly afterwards, the persisting sinus may be accompanied by the formation of granulomatous aural polyps (acute and chronic otitis media). *Cholesteatoma* is not a tumour, but consists of a granulomatous reaction containing squamous epithelium, keratin and cholesterol crystals resulting from chronic inflammation in the middle ear and mastoid. It gradually erodes the temporal bone.

There are three main causes of *deafness*—chronic otitis media, otosclerosis, and degenerative changes in the auditory nerve. Otitis media causes deafness either because the pharyngotympanic (Eustachian) tube becomes blocked by inflammatory exudate or because the ear drum is badly perforated. Otosclerosis is a condition where the oval window of the bony labyrinth becomes first increasingly vascular, and then transformed to a more spongy bone. Deafness arises when this process, which is of unknown aetiology, extends on to the fibrous annular ligament of the stapes which fits into the window. Degeneration of the auditory nerve is most likely to follow an acute viral infection, such as measles.

The Eye

The eye can become disorganized and inflamed as a result of *trauma*. It has long been known that if one eye is damaged there is a risk of serious destructive inflammation arising in the other one (sympathetic ophthalmia). It is probable that this unwelcome complication has an autoimmune reaction as its basis.

Two primary *malignant tumours* are liable to arise within the eye, with approximately equal frequency. Malignant melanoma is the one more likely to develop in adults of the older age group, arising most frequently in the choroid and detaching the retina over it as it grows. The tumour is liable to spread by way of blood stream and is a well-known cause of the appearance of delayed metastases, the liver being frequently thus involved. Retinoblastoma is the tumour which is likely to arise in early life. Most arise sporadically but some are undoubtedly hereditary. The tumour spreads preferentially along the optic nerve into the brain but may metastasize distantly outside the central nervous system being virtually the only tumour of glial origin known to be able to do this.

Cataract is an opacity of the lens and may be predominantly peripheral or central. Common causes of cataract are senility, trauma, diabetes and congenital defects which may be due to rubella infection during intrauterine life. Diabetes, in addition to causing cataracts, also results in characteristic retinal capillary microaneurysms visible through an ophthalmoscope. Haemorrhages from these aneurysms are associated with vascular proliferation extending into the vitreous and causing retinal detachment—*retinitis proliferans*. *Retrolental fibroplasia* is a condition found in premature babies exposed to an oxygen concentration of more than 40 per cent. It is caused by retinal vascular proliferation extending into the vitreous with condensation of this tissue behind the lens. *Toxoplasmosis* is an infection which is becoming recognized as a cause of choroidoretinitis and may be a congenital infection or acquired in later life (p. 64).

The *conjunctiva* is liable to many of the pathological changes which affect squamous epithelium elsewhere. Conjunctivitis is the commonest disease to occur and is due to trauma or infection. In the latter case viruses, e.g. adenovirus, are more frequent causal agents than bacteria. An important virus infection is *trachoma*, which results in a heavy lymphocytic infiltration leading to epithelial proliferation. There is vascularization of the cornea and much scarring leading to blindness.

The *orbit* may be the seat of pathological changes which reveal themselves through the eye being pushed forward (proptosis or exophthalmia). This is a well-known complication of hyperthyroidism and it is due to connective tissue oedema. There is still doubt about the cause of the oedema. It has been ascribed to the action of long acting thyroid stimulator (LATS) high levels of which arc found in primary thyrotoxicosis. However, improvement does not always accompany a fall in the level of LATS in the serum. The improvement with pituitary ablation suggests a factor from this source being involved. Proptosis can also be produced by malignant tumours, either primary or secondary, occurring in the orbital bones, paranasal air sinuses, orbital fat or optic nerve. Proptosis may be caused by a chronic fibrosing inflammatory process called pseudo-tumour of the orbit of unknown aetiology.

The Subcutaneous Tissues of the Neck

The Salivary Glands

Mumps is a virus infection to which the salivary glands, especially the parotid, are susceptible. As most cases of mumps recover little is known of the pathological change in this disease, which will also at times infect other tissues in the body, e.g. the pancreas, the testes and the brain. *Suppurative bacterial infection* may occur chiefly in the parotid gland, as a complication of other severe diseases, especially of the gastro-intestinal tract. Chronic inflammation and atrophy of the salivary glands may follow obstruction of the main duct by a *calculus*. Much of the epithelial tissue then becomes atrophic and replaced by fat and fibrous tissue. *Sjörgren's syndrome* is a cause of salivary gland enlargement. It occurs particularly in middle-aged women and is associated with a dry mouth, dry eyes and rheumatoid arthritis. The salivary and lacrimal glands become infiltrated by lymphocytes and there is atrophy of the epithelium. *Mikulicz's syndrome* is a term used to describe salivary and lacrimal gland enlargement due to a variety of causes including sarcoidosis, tuberculosis, malignant lymphoma and leukaemia.

Salivary Gland Tumours

These tumours occur predominantly in the parotid gland, the submandibular gland being the next commonest site. Tumours in the sublingual and minor salivary glands in the mouth are uncommon. By far the commonest tumour is the *pleomorphic adenoma* which occurs mainly in the parotid and is sometimes called a *mixed parotid tumour*. It is a lobulated tumour, often poorly encapsulated so that, after attempted excision, tumour remnants are left and give rise to recurrences. The tumour may be firm and glistening or mucoid. It consists of glandular and squamous epithelium in a mucoid stroma resembling cartilage, hence the term 'mixed tumour'. It is now recognized by most pathologists that this is pseudocartilage produced by myoepithelial cells surrounding the ductular epithelium. Rarely these tumours may become malignant and then develop the features of an adenocarcinoma. Three other varieties of carcinoma are found and these are relatively more common outside the parotid gland. The *cylindroma* or *adenoid cystic carcinoma* consists of cribriform nests of cells separated by strands of hyalinized connective tissue.

Mucoepidermoid carcinomas have islands of squamous epithelium containing isolated mucus-secreting cells. *Acinic cell carcinomas* are rare clear cell tumours. These three carcinomas tend to be locally recurrent and locally infiltrative, metastasizing late to cervical or preauricular lymph nodes.

Warthin's tumour (adenolymphoma) occurs almost exclusively in the parotid gland. It is derived from ductular epithelium and consists of tall columnar epithelium in an abundant lymphoid stroma. These tumours are benign.

Nerve sheath tumours arising on the facial nerve may occur in the parotid gland but other connective tissue tumours and malignant lymphomas are rare.

Branchial Cysts

These congenital cystic structures exist in the lateral aspect of the neck and are lined by stratified squamous epithelium surrounded by abundant lymphoid tissue. They are considered to develop from branchial cleft remnants, but this view has its critics.

Thyroglossal Cysts

These develop in the midline between the thyroid gland and the back of the tongue in the pathway of the embryonic thyroglossal duct. When in the upper part they are lined by squamous epithelium, when in the lower by ciliated columnar epithelium. A few thyroid acini may be present in the wall.

Lymph Nodes

Enlarged lymph nodes may frequently be palpated in the neck. Most often the enlargement is due to virus infection (glandular fever, adenovirus) or bacterial infection (*Streptococcus pyogenes*, tuberculosis). Sometimes the enlargement is due to malignant disease, such as malignant lymphoma, or secondary carcinoma.

19 The Alimentary System

The Oesophagus

Oesophagitis

Oesophagitis may result from infection, especially monilial infection spreading from the oral cavity. Hot, caustic and corrosive substances may also cause inflammation, ulceration and possibly fibrous stricture. One of the commonest causes of oesophagitis is reflux of gastric contents into the oesophagus and this has come to be appreciated as an important differential diagnosis of myocardial infarction as a cause of substernal pain. It may occur without gross anatomical disorder, but it is especially common when there is a hiatus hernia, i.e. partial herniation of the stomach through the diaphragmatic hiatus. The chronic inflammation may become complicated by ulceration of the mucous membrane, and after a time this may lead to fibrous stricture of the lower end of the oesophagus.

Achalasia

This is a disorder of motility affecting the whole of the oesophagus. Swallowing still promotes muscular activity but peristalsis is lost and the cardiac region remains tonically contracted; as a result the oesophagus empties incompletely and tends to enlarge. The tonic region does not become greatly hypertrophied. There is evidence of abnormality of the autonomic nerve fibres and ganglia in the muscle coat of the oesophagus in these cases.

Oesophageal Varices

Oesophageal varices arise in cases of portal hypertension, most frequently the result of cirrhosis of the liver. The submucous veins near the cardiac orifice of the stomach, and often for some distance above, become varicose. Such varicosities may become ulcerated and be the cause of severe haemorrhage, one of the more serious complications of portal hypertension. The lesions are hard to identify in the post-mortem room as the veins are then usually collapsed. The diagnosis is made radiologically.

Carcinoma

The oesophagus may develop squamous cell carcinoma (2 per cent of all malignant tumours). Most arise in the middle third, after which the lower third is more commonly involved than the upper. The disease is liable to arise in the older age groups with a male preponderance except where it occurs as a complication of the Plummer-Vinson syndrome, which is commoner in women. This syndrome consists of dysphagia, glossitis, achlorhydria and iron deficiency anaemia leading to the development of a post-cricoid mucosal web and eventually carcinoma. The carcinoma may project into the lumen. This projection, coupled with the fibrosis of the wall due to the infiltrating carcinoma, leads to obstruction of the lumen which is the basis of the dominant symptom, inability to swallow. The tumour infiltrates through the muscle coat of the oesophagus, and spreads readily into the mediastinum, as there is no serosal coat to delay the advancing carcinoma. Mediastinal lymph nodes are commonly involved. Carcinoma of the lower third of the oesophagus frequently spreads via the lymphatics to the lymph nodes on the lesser curve of the stomach. Carcinoma of the upper oesophagus may spread to the cervical lymph nodes. Ulceration into the mediastinum causes a serious inflammatory reaction. Death is usually as a result of inanition, pneumonia following aspiration of food being a contributory factor.

The lower end of the oesophagus, immediately before it enters the saccular stomach, is lined by gastric mucosa. Carcinomas in this area are therefore adenocarcinomas and they are indistinguishable from primary carcinomas in the gastric cardia extending into the lower oesophagus.

Adenocarcinoma may also develop from islands of ectopic gastric mucosa higher in the oesophagus.

Diverticula

Pulsion diverticula may arise as a result of herniation in the postero-lateral aspect of the hypopharynx occurring between the circular and the oblique fibres of the inferior constrictor muscle of the pharynx. The diverticulum becomes enlarged by swallowing and is filled with undigested food. *Traction diverticula* are most common in the middle third of the oesophagus due to chronic tuberculosis of the interbronchial lymph nodes leading to fibrous contraction of surrounding tissues.

The Stomach and Duodenum

The study of diffuse lesions of the gastric mucous membrane has for long been hampered because of the extensive autolysis which takes place rapidly after death. The advent of the gastric biopsy technique, added to the study of operative specimens, has made our understanding clearer.

Acute Gastritis

Acute gastritis is common in a mild self-limiting form, being produced by the ingestion of various irritants, such as alcohol, aspirin and bacterial toxins (*Staphylococcus, Salmonella*). The mucous membrane shows increased shedding of epithelium and signs of regenerative activity. A small number of inflammatory cells including polymorphs may accumulate in the lamina propria. The changes may lead to those of chronic gastritis.

Chronic Gastritis and Gastric Atrophy

Chronic gastritis is divided into two main types, chronic superficial gastritis and chronic atrophic gastritis. In the former, the thickness of the gastric mucosa is not reduced and the inflammatory reaction is confined to the superficial layers, sparing the deeper glands. This pattern is seen in chronic alcoholics and also shows an increased incidence with age. Chronic atrophic gastritis affects the body of the stomach and causes the mucosa to become thin. The chronic inflammatory reaction extends through the full thickness of the mucosa and there is atrophy of the glandular epithelium. The mucosa may show development of goblet cells in the surface layer of epithelium and Paneth cells in the glands producing a pattern of epithelium normally found in the intestine and referred to as intestinal metaplasia. This form of gastritis merges imperceptibly into gastric atrophy which is found in patients with Addisonian pernicious anaemia. Although atrophy is severe there is no inflammation. The loss of oxyntic and parietal cells from the gastric glands results in achlorhydria and absence of intrinsic factor. Antibodies to parietal cells can be demonstrated in the serum of these patients. There is often severe intestinal metaplasia which is commonly believed to lead to gastric carcinoma.

Chronic hypertrophic gastritis is not an inflammatory lesion of the stomach. It is a rare disorder in which the mucosal folds become prominent and covered with hyperplastic glands which secrete abundant mucus. The evidence suggests that this is a developmental abnormality (Menetrier's disease).

Peptic Ulcers

Peptic ulcers comprise gastric and duodenal ulcers, as well as ulcers developing after gastro-enterostomy (stomal ulcers) and those developing in ectopic mucous membrane such as in Meckel's diverticulum and in the oesophagus. On the basis of their pathology, they are divisible into acute and chronic forms.

Acute Peptic Ulcers

The true incidence of these ulcers is unknown. Only those which bleed or perforate into the peritoneal cavity can be identified clinically. Since these examples only have a short history of non-specific dyspepsia and as acute ulcers are quite common events in the post-mortem room, their incidence is probably quite high. Gastroscopy has revealed the presence of many small 'haemorrhagic erosions' in some individuals, which have been shown to heal within a few days. Acute ulcers may also take the form of larger erosions fewer in number, about a centimetre in diameter, which also can heal very rapidly without scar formation. Histologically the ulcers consist of breaches of mucous membrane with little reaction in the underlying tissue. In the smaller examples, the necrotic mucous membrane will be still *in situ* and haemorrhage will be observed to be taking place from the capillaries of the lamina propria.

The histological picture is that of a small infarct suggesting, in the absence of thrombus or embolus, that vascular spasm may be the cause. As acute ulcers may be a consequence of operation or other disturbance at the base of the brain and may follow severe burns, remotely controlled humoral or nervous mechanisms are possibly the basis of their formation.

Chronic Peptic Ulcers: Chronic Gastric Ulcer and Chronic Duodena Ulcer

Since scars or other evidence of chronic peptic ulcer can be seen in about 10 per cent of all autopsies, it is clear that this condition must be one of the commonest serious disorders to affect patients. Both gastric and duodenal ulcers are much less common in women. As with acute ulcers, some active chronic peptic ulcers will be incidental findings in the post-mortem room. Duodenal ulcer is at the present time about two or three times as common as gastric ulcer, the ratio being greater in men than in women.

Pathology. Chronic gastric ulcers occur most commonly along the lesser curve and the adjoining posterior wall. Duodenal ulcers are situated in the first part usually adjacent to the pylorus on the anterior and posterior walls. The ulcers are usually single. When two or more exist, they are most frequently observed in the same organ, but both gastric and duodenal ulcers are seen in the same patient more frequently than might be expected through chance. Apart from the fact that gastric ulcers tend to be larger, the pathological pictures presented by the two peptic ulcers are similar. They consist of sharply circular pits in the mucous membrane varying in size from a few millimetres to 3 or 4 centimetres in diameter: they are more commonly small than large. Their floors contain necrotic slough under which lie the reactive fibrous tissues typical of a chronic inflammatory process, the muscle coat having been breached. The ulcer may be shallow, or have eroded so deeply that underlying structures such as the pancreas form part of the floor.

Microscopically the ulcer floor consists of four zones. Superficially there is a purulent exudate under which is a layer of necrotic tissue. Outside the latter there is a zone of granulation tissue which merges into the outer layer of fibrous tissue. It is common to see medium-sized arteries in the ulcer floor; their lumina are usually practically occluded by endarteritis obliterans, and some in fact may contain organizing thrombi. In a proportion of cases the process of ulceration will involve the vessel wall, and, if the above regressive changes are not complete, this will lead to serious haemorrhage (haematemesis and melaena). Such eroded arteries are clearly visible to the naked eye in the ulcer floor. At the side of the ulcer, the breached muscle coat can be seen microscopically to curve upwards to meet the mucous membrane and muscularis mucosa curving downwards. The epithelium at the edge of the ulcer frequently shows atypical hyperplastic features, a reaction of epithelial cells which is common at the edge of chronic inflammatory ulcers in any situation in the body.

Progress. (1) The ulcer frequently heals. Macroscopically the site will usually be evident because of radial ridges caused by fibrous tissue which remains under the re-epithelialized floor. Microscopically, evidence that healing has begun is shown by a reduction in the amount of granulation tissue together with a spreading in from the sides of a layer of epithelium, one cell thick. Later this becomes more complicated to resemble normal lining mucous membrane. (2) Haemorrhage may result; it may be massive through erosion of an artery in the floor, or occult as a result of seepage from the granulation tissue, in which case symptoms of chronic iron deficiency anaemia may develop. A severe haemorrhage often produces a vasovagal attack, or faint, which may pass into the condition of oligaemic (surgical) shock. (3) The ulcerative process may be so vigorous that the fibrous barrier may be inadequate and incomplete, resulting in perforation into the peritoneal cavity and acute, usually generalized, peritonitis. (4) Pyloric obstruction is mainly a complication of chronic duodenal ulcer but may occasionally be produced by a pre-pyloric chronic gastric ulcer. The ulcer scarring gradually narrows the lumen of the pylorus, and oedema of the mucous membrane completes the process. Proximal dilatation of the stomach results, and this may reach considerable proportions. (5) The precise relationship between gastric ulcer and carcinoma is not clear. The incidence quoted for cancer developing in a long-standing peptic ulcer (ulcer-cancer) varies from 0 to 10 per cent, but if strict histological criteria are used, the incidence is found to be very low and nowhere near 10 per cent. Since any gastric carcinoma is liable to ulcerate, it must be distinguished from ulcer-cancer. The criteria for the latter are (a) sharply demarcated ulcer, (b) fibrosis of the muscle coat deep to the ulcer, (c) curving up of the muscular coat at the edge of the ulcer to meet the mucosa and muscularis mucosa—features of chronic peptic ulceration, (d) no carcinoma in the base of the ulcer, (e) carcinoma limited to part of the circumference of the ulcer only, (f) infiltration of the carcinoma through the muscularis mucosa. For each ulcer-cancer there are five or six ulcerated carcinomas.

Aetiology. Chronic gastric and duodenal ulcers are aetiologically quite distinct. Gastric ulcer has a greater and earlier incidence in poorer people, while the incidence of duodenal ulcer is remarkably uniform throughout the social grades of the population. This has suggested that gastric ulcers may be due in part to malnutrition, an hypothesis supported by the high incidence of gastric ulcer in parts of Asia. The tendency to develop either type of ulcer is separately inherited; relatives of patients with duodenal ulcer are more than normally liable to develop duodenal ulcers but not gastric ulcers, and vice versa. Duodenal and, to a lesser degree, gastric ulcers are unduly frequent in those of blood group O. All peptic ulcers are associated with acid secretion by gastric mucosa, but duodenal ulcers are associated with increased secretion whereas gastric ulcers have less acid secretion than normal. However, other factors must also be considered as they play a part in controlling acid secretion particularly neurogenic and psychosomatic stimuli. Hypothalamic stimulation is associated with peptic ulceration, whereas vagotomy reduces acid secretion. Conditions of stress, such as burns and brain injury may lead to acute ulceration in the stomach and duodenum. Hormonal factors are also important. Adrenal corticosteroids can cause an exacerbation of a quiescent ulcer, but they are probably not able to initiate an ulcer in a subject who would otherwise remain without one. Non-insulin secreting α-cell tumours of the pancreatic islets are sometimes associated with hypersecretion of acid and intractible peptic ulceration (Zollinger-Ellison syndrome). There is little evidence to support trauma to the gastric mucosa as being an important aetiological agent.

The pathogenesis of peptic ulcers remains obscure. It is easy to see that once the breach has occurred the secretions might help to maintain the ulceration. However, both acute and chronic ulcers heal spontaneously and acute ulcers do not usually develop into chronic ones, since they do not have the anatomical localization of the chronic lesions.

CARCINOMA OF STOMACH

Deaths from malignant disease of stomach total about 10 per cent of all deaths from all causes of malignancy. As the prognosis is among the worst of all malignant tumours, this figure probably is representative of incidence as well as death. Only malignant disease of the bronchus is a commoner cause of death in males, that of breast in females. It is a disease of middle and old age with a preponderance in lower social classes. Conditions which appear to be pre-malignant are the uncommon adenomatous polyps, chronic peptic ulcer (p. 184), and gastric atrophy (p. 182). The disease is commoner in Eastern Asia and among people of blood group A.

Macroscopic Appearance

Carcinoma of the stomach presents a wide spectrum of pathological patterns, ranging from the relatively uncommon florid polypoid lesion, through irregularly formed ulcers to ones which only flatten the mucosal surface but infiltrate widely in the wall. The latter lead frequently to a diffuse fibrosis of the wall, so that if most of the viscus is involved it becomes firm and much shrunken (the so-called leather-bottle stomach, or linitis plastica). Carcinoma originates most frequently in the pylorus and antrum (50 per cent) and on the lesser curve (25 per cent). Pyloric obstruction, as a result, is a frequent complication. When the neoplasm arises at the cardiac orifice (10 per cent) it is clinically indistinguishable from carcinoma of the lower end of the oesophagus. The tumour may be observed to have arisen in close proximity to a chronic peptic ulcer.

Microscopical Features

These are also extremely variable. The tumour is an adenocarcinoma ranging from one forming well-differentiated tubules to one which consists of separated spheroidal cells. The bulk are rather poorly-differentiated, though showing evidence of their glandular origin. The tumours are prone to produce mucus, though unexpectedly this tendency does not bear a direct relationship to the differentiation of the tumour, but rather the reverse. A common and fairly diagnostic finding is that of a spheroidal cell with its nucleus pressed to one side by a globule of mucus (signet-ring cell). The mucus production can be at times so prominent that the tumour appears gelatinous and semitransparent macroscopically (mucoid or 'colloid' carcinoma). This latter change is more conspicuous than significant. The fibrous tissue stromal reaction varies considerably. Most tumours develop a moderate fibrous stroma; those with a leather-bottle structure are extremely fibrous, and indeed it may be difficult at times to identify the carcinoma cells scattered in the fibrous tissue. Undifferentiated carcinoma sometimes occurs without much stromal reaction in which case the differentiation from malignant lymphoma, primarily involving the organ, may be difficult. The latter disease is much less common, but not outstandingly rare.

Spread

It is the rule rather than the exception that local infiltration is extensive by the time the patient presents for gastrectomy. Infiltration through the muscularis is usual, and microscopic spread is frequently far beyond the naked-eye extension. It is of interest, and probably of fundamental importance, that while spread is easy into the oesophagus, the neoplasm rarely extends into the mucosa of the duodenum, although it may spread in the muscle coat deep to the mucosa. Lymph node spread, chiefly along the lesser curvature and then into the porta hepatis, is very common. Distant blood-borne metastases also develop, and the liver is the viscus where secondary carcinoma is most frequently seen. Widespread extension to the peritoneum including the greater omentum, leading to ascites, is not an uncommon phenomenon (transcoelomic spread). Following this mode of spread secondary carcinoma is particularly prone to develop in the ovaries (Krukenberg tumours). In most cases, the development of metastases is confined to the abdomen. However an important site for metastatic tumour is the left supraclavicular lymph node adjacent to the thoracic duct. Enlargement of this node is often the first sign of gastric carcinoma.

Pyloric Stenosis

Obstruction of the stomach arises when the pylorus ceases to relax at the time the rest of the organ undergoes peristalsis. This is most likely to occur in male infants about three weeks after birth, as a congenital defect (congenital pyloric stenosis). The pyloric muscle becomes grossly hypertrophied and there are quantitative and qualitative changes in the nerves and ganglia of Auerbach's plexus in this area. In adults, pyloric stenosis is most commonly associated with a neighbouring chronic peptic ulcer or carcinoma. The first effect of the obstruction is usually increased peristalsis which can be detected clinically. Later the stomach becomes increasingly dilated. It is not difficult to appreciate that large vomits, often projectile in nature, result from this disorder.

Carcinoma of the Duodenum

Apart from chronic duodenal ulcer, gross pathological lesions in the duodenum are rare. Probably the most frequent are diverticula and adenocarcinoma. When the latter develops, a likely site is the ampulla of Vater, leading to the syndrome of obstructive jaundice.

The Jejunum and Ileum

Enteritis

It will be remembered from Chapter 9 that 8 litres of fluid reach the lumen of the intestine each twenty-four hours, and yet only 100 ml of this remains to be excreted in the faeces, the remainder having been absorbed mostly in the small intestine. It is not surprising therefore that when diffuse lesions arise in the small bowel, there should be some imbalance between fluid accumulation and removal within the bowel lumen, resulting in diarrhoea. The most common cause of diffuse lesions in the small bowel is infection, producing gastro-enteritis or enteritis, which lead to the clinical syndromes of diarrhoea and vomiting or to diarrhoea alone. In the majority of cases of gastro-enteritis the cause remains unknown, either because it has not been looked for or because the agent remains bacteriologically unidentified. Salmonellae are the commonest known aetiological agents, of which there are now 700 varieties. Other relatively common bacteria are *Staphylococcus aureus, Clostridium perfringens* (*welchii*), and some strains of *Escherichia coli*. A number of enteroviruses, such as Coxsackie and Echo viruses, have also been identified. Food-poisoning is a common way by which the organisms exert their effects; the other means is by way of cross-infection. *Staphylococcus* and *Clostridium perfringens* act in food-poisoning as a result of their pre-formed toxins being ingested. Many cases of staphylococcal food-poisoning arise following ingestion of canned foods; *Cl. perfringens* infection develops in twice-cooked meats.

Botulism is another rare but severe form of food-poisoning caused by the ingestion of the exotoxin of *Clostridium botulinum*. Canned meats are an important source of infection. The toxin produces widespread paralysis including the respiratory and pharyngeal muscles. Little is known of the infective lesions in the small intestine, because so few patients die, and those that do, develop autolytic changes in the intestine with extreme rapidity. A fulminating infection, extending to the colon, and often produced by staphylococci (pseudomembranous enterocolitis), shows great congestion and mucosal sloughing of the intestinal mucous membrane. Oral antibiotic therapy, by altering the intestinal flora and allowing the overgrowth of pathogenic organisms, is an important cause of pseudomembranous enterocolitis.

Enteric Fever

Enteric fever, caused by *Salmonella typhi* and *S. paratyphi* B (typhoid and paratyphoid fever), is much less frequent than it used to be, paratyphoid fever being the commoner and milder disease in this country. Because it affects many tissues in the body and because epidemics of the disease occur from time to time, its various manifestations need to be appreciated.

Infection is almost always due to the ingestion of the pathogenic organisms in food and drink. It is particularly in uncooked food such as salads, dairy produce and ice cream that infection is likely to be transmitted. Most of the organisms are destroyed in the acid gastric juice, but if they survive they invade the lymphoid tissue of the intestine, where thcv multiply. After an incubation period of ten days the clinical disease becomes evident as a septicaemia with a progressive rise in temperature, headache, epistaxis, bronchitis and abdominal symptoms of pain, constipation or diarrhoea. The lymphoid tissue of the ileum becomes swollen and after ten days of clinical disease, necrosis occurs. With separation of the slough, ulceration of the bowel occurs two or three weeks after the onset of the illness. The ulcers characteristically are longitudinal in the terminal ileum. Microscopically, the lymphoid tissue shows infiltration by large numbers of histiocytes but there is a paucity of polymorphs. The spleen is enlarged and soft and there are focal necroses in the liver with macrophage infiltration. Cardiac and striated muscle, especially the rectus abdominis muscle, shows focal necrosis (Zenker's degeneration). In the acute illness there is characteristically a leucopenia. Infection of the gall-bladder is common and the resulting chronic cholecystitis may be a cause of persistent infection, with the passage of live bacteria in the faeces resulting in a 'carrier state'. These people are clinically well but are a potential danger if involved in the handling of food or water. Chronic urinary carriers may result from renal infection.

Complications of enteric fever include intestinal haemorrhage from the erosion of vessels in the ulcers, or peritonitis from perforation of these ulcers. These are most likely to occur in the third week of the clinical disease. Osteomyelitis may result from chronic infection of the medullary cavity of bones. Bronchopneumonia may complicate the initial bronchitis; there may be a peripheral neuritis.

The disease is confirmed by blood culture in the first three weeks, urine culture in the second week and stool culture after the second week. Serum agglutination tests are valuable if they show a rising titre, but people who have received TAB for protection against enteric fever may show a rising titre due to a non-specific infection—'anamnestic reaction'.

Tuberculosis

Tuberculosis of the small intestine is a disease of increasing rarity due to the decline in incidence of bovine tuberculosis. The primary infection is now rare, but still presents in this country with lymph node enlargement in the ileocaecal region. These nodes may caseate and calcify, giving rise to tabes mesenterica, usually in the young. The primary focus in the intestine is not usually identified. In parts of Africa and Asia, primary ileocaeçal tuberculosis may present with a florid proliferating granulomatous inflammatory reaction simulating malignant disease (hyperplastic ileocaecal tuberculosis). Tubercle bacilli are usually plentiful in these lesions. Secondary intestinal tuberculosis most commonly follows pulmonary infection and the swallowing of tubercle bacilli. It leads to transverse ulcers in the distal small intestine. On healing these may cause stenosis. Infection may spread into the peritoneal cavity to give localized tuberculous peritonitis. Perforation of the intestinal ulcers usually gives a localized abscess as the infection is confined by the adhesions resulting from the preceding peritonitis.

Malabsorption Syndrome

The small intestine is the surface from which the essential foodstuffs are absorbed. Most are absorbed from the upper end, but some, such as vitamin B_{12}, are absorbed from the terminal ileum. Certain lesions in the small intestine will interfere with the proper absorption. Well-known results of these deficiencies include iron deficiency anaemia, megaloblastic anaemia (vitamin B_{12} and folic acid), osteoporosis and hypoproteinaemia (protein), steatorrhoea (fat), osteomalacia and rickets (calcium), beri-beri (vitamin B_1), pellagra (nicotinic acid), prothrombin deficiency and bleeding (vitamin K), xerophthalmia (vitamin A), dehydration and salt deficiency. The lesions which are known to produce these deficiencies are many. They include coeliac syndrome (idiopathic steatorrhoea), internal fistulae, blind loops of bowel giving rise to an abnormal intestinal flora, biliary obstruction, lymphatic obstruction, pancreatic failure and surgical resection of the bowel. In the coeliac syndrome, the normal villous pattern of the mucosa of the small intestine is lost, the villi fuse to give a flat mucosa or if less severe may show leaf-like villous folds. Microscopically, the villi are much shrunken, and there is increased inflammatory cell accumulation in the lamina propria. A complication of long-standing coeliac syndrome is the development of malignant lymphoma in the small intestine.

Crohn's Disease

This inflammatory process of obscure origin appears to be becoming more frequent. Its commonly used synonym, regional ileitis, indicates that the ileum is usually implicated. However, it is now appreciated that it may involve any part of the gastro-intestinal tract although the ileum is the commonest site of involvement. Most cases present in the third decade although it may occur at any age. Both men and women are affected. The inflammatory process produces 'skip lesion', i.e. inflamed portions of bowel in between normal ones. The affected bowel is thickened and firm. There are serosal adhesions and frequently fistulae between one loop of bowel and another or to the skin or bladder. Anal fistulae and perianal ulceration are common. The mucosa shows ulceration with oedematous surviving mucosa giving a cobblestone appearance. Histologically the dominant features are submucous oedema with dilated lymphatics, chronic inflammatory foci extending through the thickness of the bowel wall, some of the foci being lymphoid follicles and others granulomata containing epithelioid cells and Langhan's giant cells, but never caseation. The bowel lumen is narrowed, the mucous membrane ulcerated and fissures run deep into the bowel wall or form fistulae with neighbouring structures. The serosal surface shows chronic inflammation and oedema. Regional lymphadenopathy is associated with giant cell granulomata in the lymph nodes.

The narrowed segment of bowel is liable to produce intestinal obstruction. The ulcerated mucosa results in blood loss and iron deficiency anaemia, and the diseased terminal ileum leads to megaloblastic anaemia due to malabsorption of vitamin B_{12}. The disease is progressive for, although it is amenable surgery, recurrences are common.

Small Intestinal Obstruction

Obstruction of the *small intestine*, because of its length, its mesenteric attachment, and free movement, most frequently results from a band of connective tissue lying across it as in strangulated hernias, or because it gets twisted (volvulus). In both instances the blood supply is cut off and infarction occurs. Intestinal obstruction may be a complication of prolonged operative handling, or infection originating elsewhere in the peritoneal cavity, because of the development of the state of paralytic ileus. In newborn infants it may be due to inspissated meconium associated with the condition of mucoviscidosis (p. 217). In older children it may be due to intussusception where one portion of bowel passes into another, dragging its mesentery with it and resulting in obstruction to the blood supply and infarction of the bowel. The commonest site is the terminal ileum (intussusceptum) which passes into the colon (intussuscipiens). In children this may be due to adenovirus infection producing hyperplasia of lymphoid tissue which gets carried along the bowel lumen by peristalsis. In the large intestine, carcinoma is the commonest cause of intussusception. Inflammatory diseases such as tuberculosis or Crohn's disease may produce a stricture. Foreign bodies in the lumen may also cause obstruction. The first effect of obstruction of the small bowel is increased peristaltic activity of the viable bowel proximal to the obstruction, often detected clinically because of the increased intensity of the bowel sounds. Later the bowel will dilate, when the bowel sounds will become reduced. When peristalsis ceases in the dilated bowel, this segment now becomes a source of obstruction to the alimentary canal higher up, and this is what occurs in paralytic ileus. Small bowel obstruction is a highly dangerous state and will lead to death unless relieved. This is because the obstructed bowel is very liable to infection from the bacteria within the lumen and general peritonitis will ensue.

Meckel's Diverticulum

This congenital abnormality is found in 2 per cent of the population. It occurs about two feet from the ileocaecal valve as a true diverticulum, i.e. lined by mucous membrane and covered by muscle. It may be connected to the umbilicus by a fibrous band, in which remnants of the vitellointestinal duct may persist as a vitelline cyst. The diverticulum may produce symptoms because of the peptic ulceration which is liable to develop in the ectopic gastric mucous membrane commonly present.

Neoplasms

Neoplasms of the small intestine are rare and include argentaffinoma (carcinoid tumour), leiomyoma and leiomyosarcoma and malignant lymphoma. Apart from those in the ampulla of Vater, carcinomas are rare. Polyps may be found in the Peutz-Jeghers syndrome. These are tumour-like malformations rather than true neoplasms. Argentaffinomas arise from the Kultschitsky cells of the terminal ileum. The tumours are yellow and consist of nests of orderly cells infiltrating through the muscle coat of the bowel. The tumour may metastasize to regional lymph nodes and liver. When it does so it may give the 'malignant carcinoid' syndrome associated with the overproduction of 5-hydroxytryptamine (5–HT). This syndrome consists of attacks of skin flushing, diarrhoea and pulmonary stenosis due to endocardial fibrosis of the right side of the heart. The syndrome does not occur in the absence of extensive metastases.

The Appendix

Acute Appendicitis

This common acute abdominal emergency carried until recently a considerable mortality, as a result of the liability to general peritonitis following perforation of the inflamed organ. The seriousness of the disease is nowadays much lessened since antibiotic therapy has become available.

Macroscopic Picture

The affected part of the organ is usually oedematous and blotchy red with a fibrinous or fibrinopurulent exudate on the surface. In the more advanced cases, the wall becomes necrotic or gangrenous. Frequently the inflammation is confined to the distal half which is then sharply demarcated from the more normal proximal end. When this happens, a hardened pellet of faeces, a 'faecolith', will be seen filling the lumen of the inflamed section. The mucous membrane is ulcerated and the lumen may contain pus. In a proportion of cases, especially when gangrene supervenes, perforation of the wall occurs, with the result that the inflammation extends to the surrounding tissues, and, in some cases, to the whole of the peritoneal cavity. The contents of the peritoneal cavity have a great ability to localize infections, and, as a result, an 'appendix abscess' is a frequent end-result of perforation.

Microscopic Picture

Many inflamed appendices producing symptoms may look nearly normal macroscopically, but show evidence of infection histologically. The whole wall of the affected part shows the classical features of acute inflammation including the formation of an exudate on the surface. In gangrenous appendicitis the inflammatory exudate brings about obstruction to the blood supply so that part of the wall becomes necrotic. In the more rarely observed early cases, the inflammation will be limited to an ulcerated area of the mucous membrane and the tissues immediately beneath.

Progress

It is not known for certain whether acute appendicitis can regress spontaneously, though this is probable. Once diagnosed, surgical removal is the rule. The only certain occasion when the acute inflammation becomes chronic is after a perforation which subsequently becomes localized.

Aetiology

The lumen of the appendix is full of bacteria, including *Escherichia coli* and *Strep. faecalis* which are most often cultured from the inflamed organ. It is not surprising therefore that once the mucous membrane has become ulcerated the organ should become infected. The cause of the ulceration is less certainly known. A high proportion of inflamed appendices contain faecoliths, and when these are present the infected area is usually limited to that covering the faecolith. It is probable that muscular contraction in this area leads to ischaemic necrosis with subsequent ulceration. The mechanism is less clear in those cases without faecoliths. A possible explanation is that submucosal lymphoid hyperplasia at the proximal end interferes with effective drainage of the secretions formed in the more distal portions so that ulceration again occurs as a result of distension and ischaemia.

Following obstruction to the lumen of the appendix, the inflammation may resolve to leave a mucocoele. Rarely this lining epithelium becomes neoplastic to form a cystadenoma or cystadenocarcinoma of the appendix. Rupture of these lesions into the peritoneal cavity may result in pseudomyxoma peritonei (p. 245).

NEOPLASMS

Argentaffinoma or carcinoid tumour of the appendix consists of a small yellow nodule, usually at the distal end, and is most commonly picked up as an incidental finding in routine appendicectomy specimens. Those at the distal end rarely give further trouble but those at the proximal end are more likely to metastasize and give the carcinoid syndrome (p. 193).

The Colon and Rectum

The faeces are more fluid in the caecum than the rectum, because water is absorbed to some extent in the large bowel. Mucus secretion is more active in this section of the intestine than higher up and becomes excessive under conditions of diffuse stimulation such as in infection by dysentery organisms, in ulcerative colitis, or in cases of nervous irritability (mucous colitis).

DYSENTERY

Members of the genus *Shigella* are responsible for *bacillary dysentery* of which *S. sonnei* is outstandingly the most common in this country, the next most frequent being the organism of Flexner dysentery. Sonne dysentery is also the mildest form, producing usually only diarrhoea. The more severe variants result in the passage of increased amounts of blood and mucus also. Macroscopically the large bowel is congested and, in the severe cases, is covered with many shallow ulcers containing purulent exudate and affecting particularly the tips of the mucosal folds. Microscopically, the mucous membrane is infiltrated with inflammatory cells, polymorphs predominating in the acute cases, and lymphocytes and plasma cells in the more chronic cases.

Amoebic dysentery has been described earlier (p. 62).

Lymphogranuloma Inguinale

This venereal disease is caused by a virus of the lymphogranuloma-psittacosis group. It affects the rectum particularly in women. There is mucosal ulceration and submucosal granulomatous inflammation leading to stricture formation. The diagnosis is confirmed by the Frei test which consists of the intradermal infection of killed virus resulting in a local inflammatory reaction. The complement fixation test is more specific.

Diverticulosis and Diverticulitis

Diverticula, consisting of herniations of mucous membrane and submucosa through the muscularis (i.e. 'false' diverticula in contrast to 'true' diverticula which are pouches covered by all layers of the bowel wall and which are congenital in origin), are common in the colon, increasing in frequency with age, being uncommon under 35. They are usually multiple and most frequently located in the sigmoid colon where they form small outpushings which may extend into the appendices epiploicae between the mesenteric and anti-mesenteric taeniae. Excessive bowel contraction is considered to be an important factor in making them become larger. The muscle coat of the bowel in the affected area is grossly thickened and firm. Circular muscle fibres cause indentation of the bowel lumen. Diverticulosis is the name given to the presence of multiple diverticula, when present in the symptomless state. The mucous membrane of the diverticula is, however, liable to ulcerate, and the surrounding serous coat then becomes the seat of episodes of inflammation or diverticulitis which may lead to abdominal pain. On occasions, the ulceration is followed by stricture formation or by perforation into the peritoneal cavity. Bleeding is another important complication.

Chronic Ulcerative Colitis

This is a distressing disease affecting any age group but presenting most commonly in early adult life. It is of obscure aetiology, and leads to the passage of a large number of stools in the day usually consisting of blood and mucus. Spontaneous regression can take place, but the disease is liable to become chronic, and to require extensive surgical excision for the amelioration of the symptoms.

Macroscopic Picture

The disease may affect any part or all of the large bowel but it is usually most severe in the descending colon and rectum. Many cases appear to start in the rectum as idiopathic proctitis. In the affected areas, the whole mucosa is diseased, differing from Crohn's disease where islands of normal mucosa are interspersed in diseased areas to produce 'skip lesions'. The inflammation usually stops short at the ileocaecal valve, but where this is incompetent there may be a 'back-wash ileitis'. The affected bowel is shortened and the wall thickened with loss of normal haustrations. The mucosa is congested and covered by shallow ulcers. These rarely extend into the muscle coat and inflammation is confined to the superficial layers, unlike the transmural inflammation and deep fissures of Crohn's disease. In severe cases the neighbouring ulcers may coalesce leaving tags of surviving mucous membrane to project from the ulcerated surface. These tags may be numerous and at times show reactive proliferation, so that the bowel appears to be covered with polyps (pseudo-polyposis coli), similar to the rare hereditary condition, polyposis coli. Despite the extensive inflammation and ulceration, reactive fibrosis of the underlying wall is rare. Occasionally, fulminating cases occur in which the colon becomes grossly dilated and friable. This state of toxic megacolon carries a high mortality and surgery is difficult because of the friability of the bowel. It is in this state that perforation of the colon is most likely in ulcerative colitis. Other complications include iron deficiency anaemia, hypoproteinaemia, arthritis, skin lesions of pyoderma gangrenosum and erythema nodosum, and lastly carcinoma of the colon. Carcinoma is liable to develop in cases of long-standing ulcerative colitis, although the mucosa is usually atrophic at this time. The presence of carcinoma in the colon can often be predicted by the presence of glandular atypia on rectal biopsy. It is a wise precaution to keep long-standing cases under review for this reason.

Microscopic Picture

The mucous membrane and submucosa is congested and heavily infiltrated with lymphocytes and plasma cells whereas the muscularis usually remains clear. The mucous membrane shows varying degrees of ulceration. At the earliest stage, the ulcers are cryptic, i.e. start at the bottom of the gland tubules. In advanced cases much of the luminal surface consists of chronic inflammatory granulation tissue. When the intervening mucous membrane is polypoid, hyperplasia of the glandular epithelium will be evident microscopically.

Ischaemic (Segmental) Colitis

This is a disease affecting middle-aged and elderly patients in which segments of the colon, most commonly the splenic flexure, become stenosed. The wall is fibrosed and there is evidence of old blood in the form of haemosiderin. There are no features to suggest Crohn's disease and all the indications are that this is of ischaemic aetiology.

More florid ischaemic changes, giving infarction of the colon, may follow endotoxic shock or other major cardiovascular catastrophies.

Neoplasms

Benign Tumours

These include the various polyps of the large intestine. *Adenomatous polyps* occur most commonly in the rectum and sigmoid colon. They increase in incidence with age and they are often multiple. Adenomatous polyps consist of hyperplastic colonic or rectal mucosa thrown up into a nodule rarely more than 2 cm diameter on a narrow stalk. *Villous papillomas* in contrast are larger and instead of arising on a stalk they are broad based involving a wide area of mucosa, most commonly in the rectum. The mucosa is hyperplastic and thrown up into many finger-like projections. Transitions between these two polyps may be found and carcinoma may develop in either of the polyps. *Familial polyposis coli* is inherited as a Mendelian dominant, but the lesions do not become manifest until early adult life. The polyps are histologically similar to adenomatous polyps. Carcinoma invariably develops in the colon of untreated cases. *Metaplastic polyps* are small sessile nodules found very frequently on sigmoidoscopy. They are benign and show no tendency to malignancy. *Juvenile polyps* and *Peutz-Jeghers polyps* are not true neoplasms but are tumour-like malformations (hamartomas) of the mucosa. Juvenile polyps are often cystic. Both types of hamartomatous polyps are usually multiple. Inflammatory polyps have already been described in association with ulcerative colitis.

Malignant Tumours

The most important malignant tumour of the large intestine is carcinoma. This is one of the commonest forms of malignancy being comparable with carcinoma of the lung. However, since approximately 50 per cent of carcinomas of the large intestine are cured by surgery, the death rate for colonic and rectal carcinoma is less than that for lung cancer. The tumour is most common in older people, rectal carcinoma being about twice as common in men as in women. Colonic carcinoma does not show the same sex variation. Most of the tumours are within range of the sigmoidoscope, about half occurring in the rectum and a quarter in the sigmoid colon. Caecum and ascending colon are important but less common sites for carcinoma. Tumours of the rectum usually carry a better prognosis than those of the caecum and ascending colon because they present earlier. This is because the distal tumours frequently cause obstruction of the solid faeces, but obstruction of liquid faeces in the caecum is late. The tumour in the caecum may present as chronic iron deficiency anaemia from intestinal blood loss or it may present with an abdominal mass and right iliac fossa pain. On the left side of the large bowel, alteration of bowel habit and the passage of bright red blood per rectum are more likely presenting symptoms. Predisposing factors include intestinal polyps including familial polyposis coli and ulcerative colitis.

Macroscopic Picture

The carcinomas usually take one of three forms, polypoid tumours, ulcers with slightly raised edges or stenosing (annular) tumours.

Ulcerating tumours are much the commonest form for rectal carcinomas, whereas polypoid forms are the most frequent in the ascending colon. Stenosing tumours occur more often in the colon than the rectum. In the later stages the carcinoma completely encircles the bowel wall. Stenosing carcinomas of the colon can give rise to large bowel obstruction, the muscular wall of the bowel above becoming hypertrophied and then dilated. Such obstructed patients are not as acutely ill as those who have small bowel obstruction.

Microscopic Picture

The great bulk of the carcinomas are well differentiated adenocarcinomas, the differentiation tending to be better in the colon than the rectum. Some of the remainder are very mucoid (colloid cancer) and a few are relatively undifferentiated or of 'signet ring' cell pattern.

Spread

This is more often than not limited to the bowel wall at the time of diagnosis. Spread may be by direct infiltration which can, in the case of the rectum, extend into neighbouring structures such as the bladder. Extension to the peritoneal coat may lead to ascites or perforation with subsequent peritonitis. The regional lymph nodes are moderately frequently infiltrated at the time of operation; blood-borne metastases at distant sites, such as the liver by way of the mesenteric veins, are a relatively infrequent occurrence. A careful study has shown that the 5-year survival rate bears a direct relation to the extent of infiltration and for this purpose the Duke's classification is used. In grade 'A', the tumour is confined to the bowel wall, (98 per cent corrected 5-year survival) in grade B, there is spread into the surrounding tissues but no lymph node metastases (78 per cent corrected 5-year survival) and in grade C there is lymph node involvement (30 per cent corrected 5-year survival).

Other malignant neoplasms of the large intestine are rare but they include lymphomas, carcinoid tumours and leiomyosarcomas.

Carcinoma of the Anus and Anal Canal

Carcinoma of the rectum is about 30 times as common as carcinoma of the anus. The tumours are usually typical squamous cell carcinomas although occasionally poorly differentiated carcinomas may mimic basal cell carcinomas. These *basiloid* carcinomas should not be confused with true basal cell carcinomas that may arise in the hair-bearing skin of the anus. Squamous cell and basiloid carcinomas may spread by lymphatics both in the direction of the inferior mesenteric vein branches and to the inguinal group of lymph nodes.

Hirschprung's Disease

This is due to a congenital defect in the ganglion cells of Meissner's and Auerbach's plexus, usually in the rectosigmoid junction, and resulting in a failure of peristalsis in this area. The affected bowel is contracted but the large bowel proximal to the obstruction becomes massively dilated and requires surgical resection of the affected aganglionic segment. In adults, an idiopathic form of megacolon is seen, but here ganglion cells in the bowel wall appear normal.

Haemorrhoids or Piles

These are dilated submucosal venous channels which lie immediately below the mucous membrane in the anal canal. They are extremely common in the older age groups and are liable to give rise to recurrent slight haemorrhage especially after defaecation. The cause in most cases is obscure but the erect posture adopted by human beings and straining at defaecation are important factors in their genesis. The recent development of haemorrhoids in a middle-aged or elderly patient should always arouse the suspicion of a carcinoma in the rectum.

20 The Alimentary System (continued)

The Liver

The liver receives by way of the portal vein the blood which has drained the gastro-intestinal tract, pancreas and spleen, and after admixture with that in the hepatic artery, the blood passes via the hepatic vein almost immediately into the right atrium of the heart. It is not surprising, therefore, that the organ should frequently show degenerative changes arising as a consequence of disturbances of nutrition and circulation. Cloudy swelling, fatty change, atrophy, necrosis, fibrosis, chronic venous congestion, amyloid disease are all reactions which take place in this organ. Some have already been described in the section on general pathology, and some will come to light in the description of the specific hepatic lesions in this chapter. The liver is an organ which is capable of considerable regeneration of its parenchyma, following necrosis of the component cells due to various agents. The liver is also an important component of the reticulo-endothelial system by virtue of the Kupffer cells lining the sinus walls and others in the portal tracts. It takes part therefore in the many activities of the system; for example, haemosiderin is stored in the Kupffer cells when the supply of body iron for haemopoiesis exceeds the demand. Finally, the liver participates in haemopoiesis in the foetus, and this ability may be observed in post-natal life under abnormal conditions, such as in haemolytic disease of the newborn, and neoplastic diseases of the bone marrow.

Infections of the Liver

Viral Hepatitis

Many viral infections affect the liver. Some may cause severe liver damage whereas others cause minor non-specific degenerative changes. Important viral causes of hepatitis are yellow fever, cytomegalic inclusion disease and rubella. Infectious mononucleosis (glandular fever) is probably a viral infection which also falls into this category. However, by far the most important forms of hepatitis are those usually described as infective (epidemic) hepatitis and serum hepatitis. These are so important that the term viral hepatitis is usually taken to refer to these two diseases.

Infective hepatitis has a short incubation period (2–6 weeks); it occurs in isolated cases or in epidemic outbreaks and is spread chiefly by the faecal–oral route. *Serum hepatitis* has a long incubation period (6 weeks to 6 months) and is transmitted from one individual to another by parenteral inoculation of blood or blood products. Recent evidence indicates that this clear epidemiological separation of the two diseases is not absolute; some cases of serum hepatitis are spread by the faecal–oral route and infective hepatitis may occasionally be transmitted by inoculation. Difficulty in isolating the virus has limited progress in this field until the discovery of an antigen found in some cases of viral hepatitis. This antigen was first found in the serum of an Australian aborigine and has since been referred to as Australia antigen or hepatitis-associated antigen. It contains protein and some lipid but is different from serum β-lipoproteins. Particles of Australia antigen have been identified in the electron microscope. Unlike other viruses they do not contain nucleic acid and the antigen probably represents only the surface coat of the virus. Other particles represent antigen-antibody complexes. The evidence indicates that Australia antigen is associated with the virus of serum hepatitis, whether this is transmitted parenterally or by the faecal–oral route. Other forms of liver disease, to be discussed later, are also associated with Australia antigen implying a similar aetiological agent. Because of its association with hepatitis, Australia antigen screening tests are important for blood donors who may be suspected of transmitting viral hepatitis. These tests are also important in renal dialysis units where outbreaks of hepatitis in patients and staff are common. In Britain about 0·1 per cent of the population have Australia antigen, but in other parts of the world, particularly in Africa and S.E. Asia, the frequency is 50 to 100 times this figure. The reason for this high frequency is not known. It may represent greater faecal–oral transmission or it may be associated with tribal customs of skin scarification. The high frequency of Australia antigen also supports the view long held, that many cases of viral hepatitis escape detection because the patients are not jaundiced.

Although serum hepatitis is a more severe illness with a higher mortality than infective hepatitis, both forms of viral hepatitis have similar pathological changes. In the early stages there is centrilobular necrosis of the liver cells with bile stasis in canaliculi and bile staining of parenchymal cells. There is periportal inflammation consisting mainly of chronic inflammatory cells, lymphocytes, plasma cells and histiocytes. Similar cells and polymorphs occur in the liver lobule, particularly in association with necrotic liver cells. In severe and fatal cases, the necrosis may involve practically all the liver (massive necrosis). The liver in these cases when seen at post mortem will be small and flabby with a wrinkled capsule and a cut surface which is yellow and structureless (acute yellow atrophy). The less severe cases recover, with regeneration of parenchymal cells and restoration of normal lobular architecture. A few cases progress to chronic forms of hepatitis leading to scarring of the liver.

Other Infections

These do not occur very frequently. Infection may spread to the liver by way of the portal vein from fulminating acute inflammation in the abdominal cavity such as suppurative appendicitis giving rise to *pyaemic abscesses*. Infection may also spread by way of the hepatic artery to the liver in cases of systemic infections especially bacterial endocarditis. Acute inflammation of the intrahepatic bile ducts (acute cholangitis) may give abscesses in portal tracts (suppurative cholangitis). This is usually secondary to obstruction of large bile ducts by stones or tumour in the common bile duct or tumour in the head of pancreas. *Amoebic abscesses* occur most commonly in the right lobe of the liver. They have a ragged necrotic lining containing amoebae. Most of the necrosis is produced by cytolytic enzymes of the amoebae and inflammation is usually slight. The necrotic contents of the abscess are reddish-brown resembling anchovy sauce. *Actinomycotic abscesses* are usually secondary to infection in the region of the appendix. Multiple abscesses produce a honeycomb pattern in the liver. The lesions contain colonies of *Actinomyces israeli* surrounded by histiocytes and polymorphs. These colonies produce the characteristic sulphur granules seen in actinomycosis. *Weil's disease* is due to infection with the spirochaete *Leptospira icterohaemorrhagiae*. It is transmitted in the urine of infected rats and passes through the skin during immersion in infected water. It causes swelling of liver cells and bile stasis. Necrosis is usually slight and focal. There is also involvement of kidneys (interstitial nephritis and tubular necrosis) heart and skeletal muscle. Granulomatous inflammation may be due to tuberculosis, sarcoidosis, syphilis or liver flukes. Hyatid cysts, the cystic stage of infection by *Taenia echinococcus* has been described earlier (p. 65).

Necrosis of the Liver

Liver necrosis, apart from that associated with the infections already described, may be focal or zonal. Focal necroses are found at random throughout the liver and are a feature of typhoid fever and of diphtheria. Zonal necroses occur in relation to the liver lobule. Yellow fever produces midzonal necrosis associated with the formation of eosinophilic, hyaline, dead liver cells (*Councilman bodies*). Centrilobular necrosis is a feature of anoxic states such as chronic venous congestion or of toxic states such as carbon tetrachloride poisoning. Periportal necrosis is found in eclampsia of pregnancy and in phosphorous poisoning.

Cirrhosis of the Liver

Definition

The word 'cirrhosis' originally referred to the tawny or yellow colour of the liver common in this condition. When it was appreciated that fibrosis was a constant change, cirrhosis came incorrectly to be synonymous with fibrosis. Fibrosis is frequently the result of unimportant focal scarring or of collapse of the reticulin framework of the liver lobule, capable of resolution. Cirrhosis is an irreversible diffuse and serious disease of the liver. The confusion of terminology had led to an internationally agreed definition of cirrhosis, which specifies (1) the liver must be diffusely involved by fibrosis resulting in loss of the normal architecture though not necessarily involving every lobule; (2) liver cell necrosis must have occurred at some stage, but it may not be present at the time of histological diagnosis; (3) nodular regeneration of liver cells has occurred.

Classification. No entirely satisfactory classification is available. The two classifications most widely used are those based on aetiological and morphological criteria.

Aetiological. Some cases of cirrhosis follow an attack of viral hepatitis and others are associated with alcoholism. Cirrhosis may be due to prolonged cholestasis, haemochromatosis, Wilson's disease (hepatolenticular degeneration) or cardiac failure. There is no good evidence in man that nutritional deficiency on its own leads to cirrhosis. The largest group is that in which no aetiological agent is apparent (cryptogenic cirrhosis).

Morphological. Cirrhosis has been classified as portal (Laennec's or fine) post-necrotic (coarse) and biliary (obstructive and Hanot's). These terms are unsatisfactory because (1) portal cirrhosis implies that fibrosis originates in portal tracts, which is not always so; (2) all forms of cirrhosis, by definition, must have liver cell necrosis at some stage; and (3) biliary cirrhosis is rarely seen in a fully established state as regeneration nodules occur late. Cirrhosis may also be classified according to the size of the regeneration nodules. Micronodular cirrhosis corresponds to portal cirrhosis and is seen particularly in alcoholics. Every lobule is destroyed and the regeneration nodules are of uniform size and less than 4 mm diameter. Macronodular cirrhosis is seen in two patterns. In one every lobule has been destroyed but the regeneration nodules vary in size, often being more than 4 mm diameter. This pattern may be found in alcoholic cirrhosis after withdrawal of alcohol when continued growth of nodules causes them to become macronodular. The second pattern of macronodular cirrhosis shows coarse scarring of the liver, with large and irregular regeneration nodules, but not necessarily involving every liver lobule, so that some central veins and portal tracts may be found with their normal relationship preserved. This corresponds to post-necrotic cirrhosis and may follow viral hepatitis.

Macroscopic

The liver in portal (micronodular) cirrhosis may be small or it may be large and fatty. In post-necrotic (macronodular) cirrhosis it is usually small and coarsely scarred. On section, the regeneration nodules are seen as masses of pale liver tissue separated by fibrous strands. The liver of biliary cirrhosis is green due to cholestasis and the nodularity is very fine. If there is large-duct obstruction, the cut surface of the liver may show dilated bile ducts and the cause of the obstruction such as gallstone, stricture of the common bile duct, carcinoma of the bile duct or head of pancreas, or congenital atresia may be apparent. In haemochromatosis the liver is stained mahogany brown by haemosiderin and in cardiac cirrhosis there is evidence of long-standing passive venous congestion.

Microscopic

In fully established cirrhosis regeneration nodules are separated by fibrous tissue containing the remnants of portal tracts often with proliferating, misshapen, bile ductules. In *alcoholic* (*micronodular*) *cirrhosis*, liver parenchymal cells are often distended by fat and may contain droplets of cytoplasmic 'hyaline'. This hyaline is seen in about half the cases of alcoholic cirrhosis but may also be found rarely in other forms of cirrhosis so that it is not entirely specific. In *post-necrotic* (*macronodular*) *cirrhosis*, the large nodules may contain apparently normal liver lobules. This makes for diagnostic difficulty if needle biopsies are taken from the large nodules and contain little fibrous tissue. The presence of inflammatory cells in portal tracts and necrosis of parenchymal cells indicates continuing activity of the cirrhosis. Transition stages from active hepatitis to cirrhosis may be found. These include (1) *chronic persistent hepatitis* where the lobular architecture is preserved but portal tracts are expanded by fibrous tissue containing chronic inflammatory cells and (2) *chronic aggressive hepatitis* where the lobule is broken up by fibrous tissue extending from portal tracts to central veins. The inflammatory reaction in the latter often has a high proportion of plasma cells. Chronic persistent hepatitis may resolve, but chronic aggressive hepatitis is progressive leading in time to regeneration nodules and cirrhosis. Australia antigen (p. 203) may be found associated with this form of hepatitis.

Biliary cirrhosis may be primary or secondary. Primary biliary (Hanot's) cirrhosis occurs in middle-aged women and is believed to be an autoimmune disease. Mitochondrial antibodies are demonstrated in the serum and these react with septal bile ducts causing a granulomatous destructive cholangitis. Bile stasis is apparent in canaliculi and parenchymal cells. Portal tracts become expanded and contain abnormal ductules. There is gradual destruction of liver tissue but regeneration nodules of fully established cirrhosis are rare. These patients show clinical evidence of long-standing biliary obstruction with cutaneous xanthomata.

Secondary Biliary Cirrhosis. The features of bile duct obstruction (p. 209) are apparent. The severity of bile stasis is such that liver cells die leaving pools of necrotic bile-stained debris (bile necroses or bile lakes). There is gradual destruction of parenchyma but regeneration nodules of fully established cirrhosis are rare.

Haemochromatosis is due to abnormal intestinal absorption of iron and is seen less often in women due to their precarious iron balance during menstrual life. It may be found in post-menopausal women. There is massive deposition of iron in liver parenchymal cells, Kupffer cells lining sinusoids and in portal tracts. This leads to progressive fibrosis and cirrhosis. Other organs involved include pancreas, heart, gonads and skin. Pigmentation of the skin is due partly to melanin because of melanophore stimulation by the pituitary and partly to iron deposition around skin appendages. This pigmentation together with diabetes from pancreatic destruction have given the alternative name for this disease of bronzed diabetes.

Haemosiderosis, a disease produced by excess administration of parenteral iron, repeated blood transfusions for aplastic anaemia, or long-standing haemolytic anaemia results in haemosiderin deposition in histiocytes in many organs but is not associated with cirrhosis.

Wilson's disease (*hepatolenticular degeneration*) is caused by copper deposition in liver, brain and kidney due to a deficiency of copper-binding protein—ceruloplasmin in the blood. This results in cirrhosis, degeneration of basal ganglia in the brain, aminoaciduria and staining of the cornea (Kayser-Fleischer ring).

Cardiac cirrhosis is an uncommon consequence of long-standing passive venous congestion of the liver usually due to rheumatic or congenital heart disease. Liver damage is maximal in the centre of lobules, resulting in fibrosis in this area and link-up of one central area with another (paradoxical lobulation). Regeneration nodules of surviving liver cells results in a fine cirrhosis.

Complications

These fall into three main categories, (1) portal hypertension (2) liver cell failure and (3) tumour. Because of obstruction to the blood supply through the liver, pressure rises in the portal vein and causes dilatation of anastomotic veins in the lower end of the oesophagus (oesophageal varices) and in the anterior abdominal wall (caput Medusae). Rupture of oesophageal varices results in massive haemorrhage into the gastro-intestinal tract and is one of the major causes of death. Portal hypertension also causes splenomegaly and the enlarged spleen shows evidence of congestion and old haemorrhage resulting in brown fibrous nodules (Gamna-Gandy bodies). Splenomegaly may cause a depression of all the cellular elements in the peripheral blood (hypersplenism). Liver cell failure may manifest itself in many ways. There may be mental deterioration leading to coma due to failure to detoxify ammonia. Failure to excrete oestrogens may cause gynaecomastia, testicular atrophy, spider naevi in the skin and 'liver palms'. Failure to synthesize albumin may result in hypoproteinaemia and oedema. Hypoproteinaemia is probably also a contributory factor in producing the ascites of cirrhosis although portal hypertension and fluid retention (secondary aldosteronism) play their part (p. 80). Failure to synthesize clotting factors, notably prothrombin, and Factor VII results in coagulation disorders. This may be accentuated by increased fibrinolytic activity of blood which is found in many cirrhotic patients. Cirrhosis is a very common finding in patients with primary carcinoma of the liver. In Britain about 15 per cent of patients dying with cirrhosis have a primary liver cell carcinoma. The cirrhosis is usually macronodular in type.

Extrahepatic Obstruction

It has already been indicated that jaundice may develop as a result of intrahepatic disease, such as infective hapatitis and in some cases of cirrhosis. It also arises in those relatively uncommon cases of haemolytic anaemia when the bilirubin formed from the excessive breakdown of red cells cannot be cleared by the liver effectively. The third way in which the liver becomes jaundiced is because an obstruction develops in a large bile duct often outside the liver (extrahepatic obstruction). This may arise because (1) carcinoma of the head of the pancreas obstructs the common bile duct as it runs through that viscus (2) a gall-stone becomes impacted in the duct or (3) a stricture develops in the duct, either because of damage by an impacted stone or at previous operation or because of a primary carcinoma of the duct.

Macroscopically, the liver is usually deeply jaundiced and in the later stages the surface may be finely nodular as a result of developing biliary cirrhosis. The cut surface usually shows a very distinct lobular pattern. The bile ducts are markedly dilated above the obstruction.

Microscopically, the liver cells are filled with bile granules, and small globules and cylinders of bile (bile thrombi) appear in canaliculi between adjacent liver cells. In advanced cases large bile-stained foci of necrotic liver cells develop ('bile lakes'). The individual liver cells frequently show degenerative changes. Short stellate fibrous processes usually emanate from the portal tracts which contain an increased number of bile ducts. Inflammatory cells may accumulate in the portal tracts and round necrotic liver cell foci, but they are rarely as numerous as in hepatitis, and in contrast to the latter, usually include a number of polymorphs. Drugs such as chlorpromazine produce jaundice and give a histological picture very similar to that of early extrahepatic obstruction. This is a hypersensitivity reaction and resolves on withdrawal of the drug. Testosterone produces dose-related obstructive jaundice.

Other Liver Diseases

Neoplasms

The commonest benign neoplasm, really a congenital malformation, is a cavernous haemangioma which is quite frequently to be observed in a subcapsular position at autopsy. Other hamartomas contain bile ducts. *Metastases* are by far the most frequently observed malignant tumours and these are nearly all carcinomatous. They usually occur as multiple discrete pale grey nodules and, as the centres are liable to become necrotic being most distant from the blood supply, those which project on the surface often have depressed centres. Less commonly the malignant tumours infiltrate diffusely in portal tracts and sinuses so that the neoplastic contour is not so easily seen by the naked eye. The liver may show local chronic venous congestion and cholestasis in the neighbourhood of the nodules. *Primary liver carcinoma* can take two histological forms, one resembling liver cells (hepatoma) and the other bile ducts (cholangiocarcinoma). The nodules are often multiple, and are liable to develop in cirrhotic livers. A rapidly progressive tumour (hepatoblastoma) may arise in infancy similar to the commoner primitive tumour of renal origin (nephroblastoma or Wilms' tumour).

The Bile

The liver secretes approximately 800 ml of bile per day. It contains bile acids, bile pigments, mainly bilirubin, cholesterol and mucin. The gall bladder concentrates bile four to ten times by absorption of water. Bile salts play an important part in the absorption of fats by emulsifying triglycerides. In this way they also assist in the absorption of calcium and fat soluble vitamins (A, D and K). They also assist in the activation of proteolytic enzymes. Bile is the main route of excretion of certain metabolites of drugs and hormones, heavy metals, poisons, bile pigment and cholesterol from the body.

Only 80 per cent of the bile pigment is derived from the haemoglobin of broken-down red cells; the remainder comes from an unknown source, probably other haem pigments as in muscle. Haemoglobin breaks down in the reticulo-endothelial system to haem and globin. The latter is re-metabolized. The haem forms an iron-containing fraction, haemosiderin, which is conserved by the body, and bilirubin, which is insoluble in water, becoming attached to plasma albumin on its way to the liver. The bilirubin becomes detached from the albumin and conjugated with glucuronic acid in the liver cell, and the resultant water-soluble glucuronide conjugate is passed out into the bile. When the bile reaches the intestine, it is converted by bacteria to stercobilinogen (urobilinogen). Some of this, on oxidation to stercobilin (urobilin), pigments the faeces. The remainder is reabsorbed from the intestine and passes into the liver to be re-excreted. The liver 'threshold' is higher for urobilinogen than for bile, so that when it is mildly damaged, or when an excessive load of urobilinogen is presented to it, there is delay in re-excretion of the urobilinogen, and some of the excess passes over into the urine at a time when the liver still excretes bile completely. The renal 'threshold' for albumin-bound bilirubin is much higher than for conjugated glucuronide, with the result that the former never appears in the urine.

Jaundice

The commoner forms of jaundice fall into three main groups: (a) haemolytic jaundice, (b) parenchymatous (intrahepatic) jaundice, and (c) obstructive (extrahepatic) jaundice.

(a) *Haemolytic Jaundice*

In haemolytic jaundice excessive albumin-bound bilirubin is present in the plasma as the result of the increased breakdown of red cells. The renal threshold is not exceeded so no bilirubin appears in the urine. The increased amount of bilirubin is sometimes not completely excreted by the liver as quickly as the normal amount is, so that jaundice may appear. Nevertheless the amount of bilirubin excreted is always greater than normal so that more stercobilinogen (urobilinogen) forms in the intestine and is reabsorbed into the blood. This is in excess of the powers of the liver to re-excrete it, so urobilinogen appears in the urine.

(b) *Parenchymatous Jaundice*

This falls into two categories. In the first there may be failure to transport bilirubin from the serum to the conjugation site in the liver cell. This is seen in viral hepatitis and a familial form of jaundice known as Gilbert's disease. The second category is failure to conjugate bile within the liver cell. This is seen in premature infants and accounts for 'physiological jaundice'. In these conditions the liver fails to secrete all the bilirubin but some becomes conjugated and 'regurgitates' into the blood stream. In viral hepatitis this becomes greater the more severe the damage. Bilirubin, therefore, appears in increasing amounts in the urine.

(c) *Obstructive Jaundice*

This arises as a result of intrahepatic cholestasis (Dubin-Johnson familial jaundice, chlorpromazine jaundice) or extrahepatic jaundice due to carcinoma of the pancreas or bile duct, gall-stone in the bile duct, or stricture of the duct. Less and less bilirubin is excreted into the intestine as the jaundice progresses, so the urobilinogen reabsorbed falls away and none ever appears in the urine. The retained bile in the liver regurgitates into the blood stream, and thus appears in the urine in increasing amounts with increasing duration and completeness of obstruction.

The Gall-bladder

Gall-stones

Gall-stones are extremely common being found in about a quarter of all routine post-mortems being much commoner in women than in men. The mechanisms leading to their development are still largely obscure. The old-established concept that most stones develop through infection is not proven. They arise through the precipitation of some of the three main ingredients of bile, bile pigment, cholesterol, and calcium salts, either because one or more of these components is in excess, or because there is altered absorption by the gall-bladder of water and some of the other constituents of the bile. There are three well-recognized types. (1) *Mixed stones*. These are much the commonest, and most important clinically. They are faceted, always multiple, and are composed of a mixture of bile pigment, cholesterol, calcium salts, and a protein matrix derived from the lining epithelium. They are shiny and deep greenish brown, the surface frequently being harder than the core which is laminated and shows varying pigmentation. The gall-bladders containing them are usually the seat of chronic inflammation. (2) *Pigment stones*. These stones are multiple, small, hard, rounded or nodular, and sometimes exist in the form of sand. They are black or dark green in colour, being composed chiefly of bile pigments, with a matrix of organic material and a variable amount of calcium. They occur when the amount of bile pigment is relatively high and therefore develop chiefly in cases of long-standing haemolytic anaemia. (3) *Cholesterol stones*. These stones are usually single, averaging 1–2 cm in diameter, are pale brown in colour, finely nodular on the surface, and on section show a radially disposed crystalline texture. A shell of calcium pigment may be deposited on the surface when the gall-bladders are inflamed (*combination stone*). The gall-bladders may frequently, however, be thin walled, and the mucous membrane be studded with fine creamy flecks, due to the presence of histiocytes containing fatty material (cholesterosis or 'strawberry' gall-bladder). Cholesterol is held in solution in the bile by the bile acids, and any factor which tends to increase the concentration of cholesterol or decrease that of the bile acids will favour the formation of these stones. Examples are, for the former, obesity, high fat diet, diabetes and pregnancy, for the latter, inflammation of the gall-bladder wall, bile stasis and liver disease.

Natural History of Gall-stones

The clinical manifestations of gall-bladder disease are nearly all the result of the development of gall-stones. Gall-stones tend to be silent clinically unless they migrate into the neck of the gall-bladder or into the common bile duct. In the former case, the retained bile may lead to irritation of the gall-bladder wall and secondary infection giving *acute or chronic cholecystitis*. If the infection is more severe, the gall-bladder may become gangrenous and perforate or result in an empyema of the gall bladder. Inflammation may lead to the formation of fistulae into surrounding structures, notably the small intestine. Large stones passing through these fistulae may cause intestinal obstruction and gall-stone ileus. Obstruction to the neck of the gall-bladder results in absorption of pigment from the retained bile and accumulation of mucus—a mucocele of the gall-bladder. Most examples of carcinoma of the gall-bladder develop in those containing stones and showing changes of chronic cholecystitis. The passage of gall-stones down the common bile duct may be silent or may produce symptoms of pain with intermittent obstructive jaundice. If unrelieved, this may give ascending cholangitis and biliary cirrhosis.

Acute Cholecystitis

This, in isolation, is relatively uncommon. It is more frequently seen as an exacerbation of chronic inflammation. There is evidence that the inflammation is initially not bacterial, for in the early period the bile is sterile. However, after 24 hours, infection is superimposed on the chemical inflammation. Macroscopically the gall-bladder shows all the features of acute inflammation with ulceration of the mucous membrane and the development of pus in the bile. Necrosis and perforation may result in peritonitis.

Chronic Cholecystitis

This is much more commonly observed. The gall-bladder is shrunken and pale grey, with fibrous adhesions on the surface. On section the wall is greatly thickened, and the mucous membrane pale olive green, pitted and somewhat velvety. Microscopically the normal papillary mucous membrane is considerably flattened and may be absent in places. There is a great increase of fibrous tissue in the wall, chiefly located outside the muscle coat. A variable amount of chronic inflammatory cell infiltration is present. The mucous membrane is liable to herniate through the loose muscularis to form the so-called Rokitansky-Aschoff sinuses. These may ulcerate, and the bile in the lumen may thus add to the chronic inflammatory reaction in the wall. The arteries in the wall show evidence of endarteritis obliterans.

Gall-stone Impaction in the Common Duct

This is the commonest cause of extrahepatic biliary obstruction, and the jaundice is classically associated with pain with or without intermittent fever. In a proportion of cases, however, the jaundice is symptomless. The bile duct is dilated above the obstruction. In a minority of cases, acute purulent inflammation of the proximal branches may develop (acute cholangitis). Stones impacted in the ampulla of Vater may be associated with acute pancreatitis.

Tumours of the Gall-bladder and Bile Ducts

Papillary adenomas may occasionally develop in the gall-bladder. Carcinomas form about 1 per cent of all malignant tumours. They occur mostly either at the fundus or the neck and tend to infiltrate locally into the adjacent liver. Metastases to the regional lymph nodes are common. Most are adenocarcinomas of varying differentiation but sometimes metaplastic squamous carcinomas develop. Carcinomas of the bile duct are of the same order of frequency, are also adenocarcinomas and either cause stricture of a main duct or present as an intrahepatic tumour.

The Pancreas

Diabetes Mellitus

This disease is due to a relative or absolute lack of insulin and is the commonest disease implicating the pancreas. The causes have already been mentioned (p. 34). The pancreas is usually normal macroscopically and in half the cases the islets appear normal microscopically. In the remainder there are varying degrees of hyalinization of the islets or hydropic degeneration of the β cells. Because of the insulin lack there is impairment of glucose metabolism and increased gluconeogenesis from fat and protein, resulting in hyperglycaemia, ketosis, glycosuria and ketonuria. The presence of ketosis is of more serious import than the glycosuria or hyperglycaemia, for it indicates the presence of metabolic acidosis and when severe gives rise to diabetic coma. The more important manifestations of diabetes include the tendency to infections, including pulmonary tuberculosis, pyelonephritis and papillitis necroticans in the kidney, nodular glomerular sclerosis (Kimmelstiel-Wilson kidney) which may cause the nephrotic syndrome, atherosclerosis and resultant ischaemic changes in brain, heart, kidney or limbs, retinal microaneurysms and retinitis proliferans in the eye, cutaneous necrobiosis lipoidica, peripheral neuritis and obstetrical complications associated with large babies or eclampsia. Diabetic women have an increased tendency to develop endometrial carcinoma.

Carcinoma of the Pancreas

This forms about 4 per cent of all malignant tumours, occurring rather more frequently in men than women and in the older age groups. Three-quarters arise in the head and by local spread form an important cause of silently progressive jaundice of extrahepatic origin. The less common body and tail carcinomas are liable to present either by a flitting thrombo-phlebitis or by way of metastases, as the primary site is undetectable clinically. Macroscopically the carcinoma usually forms a hard pale grey nodule with ill-defined borders. Microscopically it is an adenocarcinoma, usually in abundant fibrous stroma, and may be either predominantly ductular and perhaps mucus secreting or mainly of acinar pattern. It spreads into surrounding structures of which the common bile duct and vertebrae are of greatest clinical importance. Lymphatic spread occurs to lymph nodes around the head of the pancreas, along its upper border and in the porta hepatis. Blood spread to the liver is common and transcoelomic spread may give malignant ascites. Secondary carcinoma in the pancreas is a more frequently observed tumour than the primary tumour.

Pancreatitis

This may occur in acute and chronic forms. *Acute interstitial pancreatitis* develops as a complication of mumps, but little is known of the microscopical lesion in this instance, as nearly all cases recover spontaneously. *Acute haemorrhagic pancreatitis* is a well-recognized cause of an acute abdominal emergency, which is much more frequently diagnosed than substantiated. It is brought about by digestion of the organ and surrounding peritoneal fatty tissue by its own powerful enzymes. The mechanism of the release of the enzymes is obscure, but appears to be associated with a rise in intraductular pressure. There may be a gall-stone impacted in the ampulla of Vater or there may be a stricture of the pancreatic duct. Attacks frequently follow large meals and are more common in alcoholics. Less commonly the initiating factor may be vascular, either atheroma or polyarteritis nodosa, causing ischaemic necrosis of the gland and release of digestive enzymes. The pancreas is swollen and haemorrhagic. Creamy yellow flecks of fat necrosis may be seen in the surrounding fat. Microscopically, the pancreas is largely autolysed and areas of haemorrhage are present with some exudation of polymorph leucocytes. The latter are usually few in number as most of the inflammation and necrosis are chemical. High levels of serum amylase confirm the diagnosis. Acute pancreatitis is a serious disease with a high mortality. A few cases recover but they may be left with a pseudocyst of the pancreas consisting of incompletely organized blood clot and fat necrosis. *Chronic pancreatitis* is another disease of obscure aetiology. It appears to follow repeated minor attacks of acute pancreatitis and is particularly associated with alcoholism. Some cases may also follow obstruction of the pancreatic duct or ampulla of Vater by carcinoma or calculus. The pancreas feels diffusely firm or hard and may suggest carcinoma. The histological picture is one of glandular atrophy, initially with surviving islets of Langerhans but later these also atrophy, to be replaced by fibrous tissue. There may be infiltration of the gland by chronic inflammatory cells. Haemochromatosis (p. 208) may also give diffuse fibrosis of the pancreas, but this is associated with heavy deposition of iron.

Fibrocystic Disease

Fibrocystic disease produces a pathological picture in the pancreas similar to that of chronic pancreatitis except that the surviving ducts are usually cystic and contain inspissated mucin. This forms part of a systemic disease involving mucus secretion in ducts in the pancreas, lungs and liver; it also involves sweat glands and salivary glands. The disease is more appropriately referred to as *mucoviscidosis*. It is hereditary and occurs in about 0·2 per cent of infants. In neonatal life it may present as intestinal obstruction due to inspissated meconium in the gut—meconium ileus. Later, it becomes manifest as malabsorption due to pancreatic failure. These children also develop bronchiectasis with recurrent respiratory infections, and chronic biliary obstruction leading to cirrhosis. There is excessive secretion of sodium and chloride by sweat glands and salivary glands. The disease is considered by some to be due to an abnormality of mucolytic enzymes but others regard it as due to an abnormal mucin.

Pancreatic Cysts

Retention cysts in the pancreas may be associated with duct obstruction as found in mucoviscidosis. *Congenital cysts* are usually larger, and lined by duct epithelium; there may also be cysts in the kidney and liver. A syndrome of cerebellar angiomata with pancreatic and renal cysts is known as Lindau—von Hippel disease. *Pseudocysts* do not have an epithelial lining. They consist of old blood and cellular debris surrounded by fibrous tissue, the result of previous acute haemorrhagic pancreatitis or trauma. *Neoplastic cysts* may be benign or malignant. These cystadenomas and cystadenocarcinomas are mucus secreting and are similar to the corresponding mucinous cysts in the ovary.

Islet Cell Tumour

Islet cell tumour is rare, usually small, single, and benign, but may sometimes be multiple. It is of interest because it commonly consists of β cells and secretes excessive amounts of insulin leading to spontaneous hypoglycaemia. Some tumours, however, consist of α cells and these may be associated with diarrhoea and intractable peptic ulceration of the stomach or duodenum (Zollinger-Ellison syndrome). The tumours look similar, microscopically, to carcinoid tumours. About 10 per cent of these tumours are malignant and metastasize by the lymphatics to local lymph nodes and by the blood stream to the liver.

Further Reading

Sherlock, S. (1968) *Diseases of the Liver and Biliary System.* 4th edn. Oxford, Blackwell.

21 The Urinary Tract

The Kidneys

Disease of the kidneys comes to the notice of clinicians because of the effects of (a) functional failure, (b) hypertension, (c) infection and (d) malignant disease. Functional failure may be due to pre-renal, renal, or post-renal causes. Pre-renal factors include cardiac failure, dehydration and surgical shock. Renal factors usually follow one of a few well-defined clinical patterns: (1) Acute renal failure, with oliguria or anuria. This may follow mismatched blood transfusion, severe crush injuries or poisoning with drugs. (2) Chronic renal failure with the development of chronic uraemic symptoms. This is most commonly the result of chronic glomerulonephritis and chronic pyelonephritis. (3) Acute nephritic syndrome characterized by oedema, haematuria, oliguria, proteinuria and hypertension. (4) The nephrotic syndrome consisting of severe oedema, proteinuria, hypo-albuminaemia and hypercholesterolaemia. This may arise as a result of a number of disease processes which can only be distinguished by renal biopsy. Post-renal factors causing functional failure include ureteric or urethral obstruction, the latter most commonly due to prostatic hyperplasia. The kidneys may fail as a result of damage by essential hypertension, or intrinsic kidney disease may be the underlying cause of the hypertension such as happens with chronic glomerulonephritis and pyelonephritis. The role of the kidneys in the causation of hypertension has already been considered (p. 145). Carcinomas of the renal parenchyma and renal pelvis, Wilms' tumour, secondary carcinoma, malignant lymphoma and leukaemia are the malignant diseases likely to involve the organ.

GLOMERULONEPHRITIS

Nomenclature: the term glomerulonephritis implies inflammation of glomeruli as seen in acute proliferative glomerulonephritis. However, there are so many features in common with other forms of non-inflammatory glomerular disease that the term glomerulonephritis is usually taken to include all forms of renal disease which principally affect glomeruli. This disease may affect all or only some glomeruli. If all are involved it is generalized and if some involved and others spared it is focal. If the whole glomerular tuft is involved it is diffuse but if only part of the tuft is affected it is segmental.

The terms acute nephritis (acute nephritic syndrome) and nephrotic syndrome refer to clinical features of glomerular disease but they do not indicate the nature of the underlying pathological processes. Glomerulonephritis is conveniently divided into proliferative and membranous forms. Ellis Type I nephritis corresponds with acute proliferative glomerulonephritis, Ellis Type II nephritis includes membranous glomerulonephritis with other causes of the nephrotic syndrome.

Proliferative Glomerulonephritis

The most typical history of this disease is of a child or young adult who suffered from an upper respiratory infection due to β-haemolytic streptococci 2–3 weeks prior to the development of acute nephritic syndrome. The oedema is typically facial and most noticeable around the eyes. Haematuria may be slight, producing a smoky haze or it may be gross, the urine then being dark brown, the colour of Coca Cola. Proteinuria is variable but infrequently exceeds 5g/24 hr. There are granular and cellular casts in the urine. Oliguria may be severe, and in some cases there may be anuria. Hypertension is of rapid onset and may cause cardiac failure or hypertensive encephalopathy.

Not all cases fit into this typical picture. Older adults may be affected. The preceding infection may be due to other organisms, or it may be undetectable. Proliferative glomerulonephritis may also be due to other diseases such as bacterial endocarditis, Henoch-Schönlein purpura, polyarteritis nodosa and disseminated lupus erythematosus. In the latter diseases glomerular involvement is more often focal and segmental.

In the typical case, the kidney is swollen and congested, the glomeruli standing out on the cut surface. Microscopically the glomeruli are all strikingly enlarged, filling the urinary space within Bowman's capsule. The tuft is hypercellular due to infiltration with neutrophil polymorphs and proliferation of capillary endothelial cells, visceral epithelial cells and mesangial cells which lie in the core of the tuft. In the early stage there is vascular congestion as would be expected in any acute inflammatory reaction. Later, as endothelial cell proliferation increases, the capillaries become narrowed and bloodless. The impairment of blood flow through the glomerular tuft diminishes the flow through the efferent arteriole to the tubules, resulting in degenerative changes of cloudy swelling in these tubules. Protein may be taken up from the lumen by the proximal tubular cells and appear as hyaline droplets within their cytoplasm.

Most of these patients recover without detectable residual renal damage. Children have a better prognosis especially when the disease can be shown to be due to β-haemolytic streptococci. In these, over 95 per cent recover compared with only 80 per cent in adults. A few die in the acute phase as a result of cerebrovascular accident or cardiac failure due to hypertension, or they die from acute renal failure. Of the remainder, especially in adults, some run a rapid progressive downhill course with death occurring 3–6 months later in chronic renal failure often with accelerated (malignant) hypertension. Others apparently recover apart from slight persistent proteinuria, but these eventually develop either the nephrotic syndrome or chronic renal failure, years later. The rapidly progressive cases usually have more severe haematuria and oliguria in the acute phase. The glomeruli, in addition to the changes already described, show proliferation of capsular epithelial cells forming epithelial crescents. There is progressive sclerosis of glomerular tufts with adhesions between the tuft and the capsule. Tubular atrophy becomes more severe and there is interstitial fibrosis and chronic inflammation. There may be superimposed histological changes of malignant hypertension. Of the more slowly progressive cases, some show a pattern of *membrano-proliferative glomerulonephritis*. In these, mesangial cells proliferate and extend from the core of the tuft around the capillary wall separating endothelial and epithelial cells. Mesangial cells produce an extracellular matrix similar to basement membrane and this is deposited adjacent to the endothelial cells increasing the thickness of the capillary wall. These cases are associated with low levels of serum complement. In time there is progressive glomerular sclerosis leading to chronic renal failure. Many of these cases pass through a nephrotic phase.

It is now believed that typical cases of proliferative glomerulonephritis are a manifestation of Type 3 hypersensitivity (p. 89) with the deposition of antigen-antibody complexes in glomerular capillary walls. These deposits can be seen on electron microscopy as 'humps' on the epithelial side of the basement membrane and they can be shown by immunofluorescence to contain 'lumpy-bumpy' deposits of IgG and complement. In Africa, glomerulonephritis may be associated with malaria and the antibody deposited in the basement membrane in these is more commonly IgM. Occasionally antibodies are found which react with glomerular basement membrane. This gives a linear pattern of immunofluorescence as seen in Goodpasture's syndrome—glomerulonephritis and haemorrhagic pneumonitis. In these cases there is cross-reaction of antibody with alveolar and glomerular basement membranes.

Nephrotic Syndrome

There are many causes of the nephrotic syndrome of which proliferative and membrano-proliferative glomerulonephritis have already been considered. Other causes include idiopathic membranous glomerulonephritis, minimal change lesion (foot process disease), diabetic glomerulosclerosis, amyloidosis, disseminated lupus erythematosus and renal vein thrombosis. *Membranous glomerulonephritis* affects adults more commonly than children and gives rise to the nephrotic syndrome without a history of preceding infection. The oedema may result in effusions into the peritoneal, pericardial and pleural cavities. Proteinuria exceeds 5g/24 hrs and because the liver is unable to synthesize albumin at a sufficient rate to replace this loss the serum protein levels fall. The loss of protein in the urine is usually unselective so that large molecules of globulin are lost with small molecules of albumin. Macroscopically the kidneys are large and pale and on section may show linear deposits of lipid in the cortical tubules. Microscopically the glomerular capillary walls become thickened due to deposition of protein on the epithelial surface of the membrane which, with silver stains, has a spiked outer border, the gaps between the spikes representing unstained deposits of protein. Immunofluorescence shows this protein as 'granular' or 'lumpy-bumpy' deposits of IgG. The deposits can be seen in the electron microscope which also reveals that the visceral epithelial cells have lost their foot processes and are smudged on to the basement membrane. The glomerular tuft gradually becomes avascular as the capillary wall thickens. Eventually glomerulosclerosis and tubular atrophy develop giving a pattern of chronic glomerulonephritis similar to that resulting from proliferative glomerulonephritis.

Minimal change lesion occurs relatively more commonly in children with the nephrotic syndrome. The macroscopic appearance of the kidney is similar to that with other causes of the nephrotic syndrome. Histologically the tubules are laden with fat but glomeruli show no changes and there are no deposits in the tuft. It was long believed that this was a tubular disease (lipoid nephrosis) but electron microscopy has revealed that there is fusion of foot processes of visceral epithelial cells in the glomerular tuft in every case. The proteinuria is usually selective so that albumin is lost but the larger globulin molecules are retained. Most of these cases respond well to steroid therapy.

Diabetic glomerulosclerosis takes two forms. The diffuse form results in uniform thickening of glomerular basement membranes and the nodular form (Kimmelstiel-Wilson kidney) shows nodules of mesangium in the peripheral parts of the core of the tuft. Both forms are associated with the nephrotic syndrome.

Amyloidosis commonly involves the kidney. Amyloid may be deposited around tubules and arterioles, but it is in the glomerular tuft that it results in heavy proteinuria. The amyloid infiltrates the capillary basement membrane and results in fusion of foot processes of visceral epithelial cells.

Disseminated lupus erythematosus is one of the causes of focal proliferative glomerulonephritis. In addition there may be glomerular basement membrane thickening due to the deposition of immunoglobulins, complement and fibrin. The bright eosinophilia of the fibrin outlines the capillary wall and gives the 'wire loop' appearance typical of this condition. Haematoxylin bodies corresponding to the inclusions of LE cells, may be found in sections of these kidneys.

Renal vein thrombosis may give the nephrotic syndrome but in some cases the thrombosis may be secondary to renal disease, notably amyloidosis, which itself may cause the nephrotic syndrome. The appearances in the kidney in renal vein thrombosis are very similar to those of membranous glomerulonephritis.

Chronic Glomerulonephritis

This disease results in one of the forms of contracted granular kidney. The organ is smaller and paler than normal, and the capsular surface is finely and irregularly nodular, the capsule being adherent in places. The normal corticomedullary pattern of the cut surface becomes obliterated and the cortex is thinned. The renal arteries may appear prominent. Histologically there is usually a striking reduction in the number of glomeruli, and the surviving ones are, to varying degrees, sclerotic. Most of the tubules will have disappeared, the remainder being atrophic and sometimes dilated. There is a considerable increase of interstitial fibrous tissue, with some chronic inflammatory cells. The arterioles and arteries may show in addition features of benign or malignant hypertension.

PYELONEPHRITIS

Pyelonephritis is more liable to occur when there is urinary stasis, *Escherichia coli, Streptococcus faecalis* and *Staphylococcus aureus* being the most likely organisms involved. In *acute pyelonephritis*, the pelvis of the kidney is congested and hyperaemic and, later, purulent streaks can be seen to radiate from it into the medulla and cortex. Abscesses may develop and coalesce in the severe cases. The kidneys are frequently only focally involved. The infection may reach the kidney by the blood stream or it may ascend the ureter.

Chronic pyelonephritis is an important cause of hypertension. The changes in the kidney are similar to those of ischaemia so that the clinical diagnosis is dependent on the demonstration of microorganisms in the urine exceeding 100 000 per ml and of a urinary leucocyte count exceeding 400 000 per hour. The most common infecting organism is *E. coli*. The kidneys are unequal in size with coarse scars and small cysts. There is reduction of cortical tissue and loss of demarcation of cortex and medulla. The renal papillae are blunt and the calyces dilated. Histologically there is glomerulosclerosis, periglomerular fibrosis, tubular atrophy, the dilated tubules containing protein casts and giving an appearance similar to that of thyroid colloid, interstitial fibrosis, chronic inflammation, and arterial changes of hypertension. The renal pelvis also shows chronic inflammation. There may be polymorph leucocyte infiltration of tubules and interstitium if the disease is active.

Papillary Necrosis

This is an important complication of phenacetin therapy over many years. There is avascular necrosis of the renal papillae which are shed in the urine, giving rise to impaired renal function. Papillary necrosis may also be a complication of acute pyelonephritis especially when this complicates diabetes mellitus or urinary obstruction.

Renal Tuberculosis

The organ becomes infected by way of the blood stream and progressive disease more frequently involves one kidney than both. It may be a complication of miliary tuberculosis in which case the small grey nodules can be seen throughout the renal parenchyma or a focal caseating lesion may be found. Focal lesions usually arise near the corticomedullary junction but spread to involve the renal pelvis giving tuberculous pyelonephritis. Obstruction to the ureter by granulomatous inflammation leads to tuberculous pyonephrosis. The histological features are typical of tuberculous granulomata. The lesions may heal, leaving fibrosis or calcified scars. Tuberculous pyonephrosis may destroy the whole renal parenchyma leaving a fibrous renal capsule surrounding caseous material—autonephrectomy. Infection commonly spreads to involve the ureter, bladder, prostate and epididymis.

Hydronephrosis

This may be unilateral or bilateral. Unilateral hydronephrosis is usually associated with ureteric obstruction which may be due to congenital stenosis at the pelvi-ureteric junction, or it may follow scarring of the surrounding tissues, tumour in the wall, or calculus in the lumen. Bilateral hydronephrosis may be due to external pressure on the ureters associated with tumour or retroperitoneal fibrosis; it may be due to tumour of the bladder or to obstruction at the bladder neck (prostatic hypertrophy) or urethra (gonococcal stricture). Hydronephrosis may involve the pelvis chiefly (extrarenal hydronephrosis) or the calyces as well (renal hydronephrosis). With increasing degrees of hydronephrosis, the renal parenchyma becomes increasingly stretched and its blood supply increasingly obstructed, so that the nephrons undergo replacement fibrosis. The kidney thus becomes progressively less able to excrete urine and ultimately renal failure (uraemia) follows. This result of urinary obstruction is complicated in many instances by infection (cystitis and pyelonephritis), which is very liable to occur whenever urine becomes stagnant in the urinary tract.

Renal Calculi

These exist in three common forms (a) uric acid, (b) calcium oxalate, and (c) calicum phosphate. The two former arise in acid urines and the latter in alkaline ones. Calculi develop as a result of precipitation of the corresponding salt when this is in excess in the urine. Calcium oxalate stones are laminated, hard and spiky or nodular. Calcium phosphate stones are larger and chalky, sometimes forming a cast of the renal pelvis (staghorn calculi). They often develop after infection with urea-splitting organisms. Uric acid stones are the least common, often yellow and smooth or nodular and are chiefly metabolic in origin. They are liable to be laminated on section. Rarely stones may be composed of amino acids. The radiological demonstration of renal calculi may be the first evidence of the existence of primary hyperparathyroidism but this accounts for less than 5 per cent of all urinary stones. Small calculi passing down the ureter cause renal colic, but larger calculi which are too big to enter the ureter are more likely to present with haematuria. Long-standing calculi in the renal pelvis may cause squamous metaplasia of the lining epithelium. Bladder calculi usually originate in the kidney but phosphate calculi may arise in the bladder.

Renal Cysts

Renal cysts may be solitary or multiple. Small cysts are common in scarred kidneys but the important form of cystic disease is congenital polycystic kidney. Microdissection has shown that the cystic change may occur at different levels in the nephron but in contrast to previous teaching, there is no failure of link-up of tubules derived from the metanephric duct with those derived from the metanephric ridge. Four patterns are recognized of which one commonly gives bilateral polycystic kidneys and another gives unilateral or partial polycystic disease. Of the remaining two types, one is fatal in neonatal life and the other is associated with intrauterine lower urinary tract obstruction. The common type associated with bilateral polycystic kidneys is familial and there is cystic change in other organs such as liver and pancreas. Polycystic disease may present clinically in infancy or early childhood as an abdominal mass or uraemia. They also present in middle adult life with uraemia, hypertension, haematuria and an abdominal mass. There may be 'berry aneurysms' on the cerebral arteries causing subarachnoid haemorrhage.

Cortical Necrosis

Bilateral symmetrical cortical necrosis is a rare complication of obstetric shock, endotoxic shock or severe dehydration in infants. The mechanism is not clearly understood but two factors seem to be of importance. There may be shunting of blood through juxtamedullary glomeruli so that the cortex is deprived of blood or there may be intravascular thrombosis in small capillaries and arterioles, seen particularly in glomeruli. This thrombosis can be produced experimentally by the repeated intravenous injection of endotoxin (Shwartzman reaction). The cortex is infarcted and there is acute renal failure which is usually fatal.

Tubular Necrosis

This is more common than cortical necrosis and is seen following renal transplantation, shock, crush injury or incompatible blood transfusions. Grossly the kidneys may be slightly enlarged and pale. Histologically the lower nephron contains many pigment casts and the lining epithelium is lost. Tubular epithelium may regenerate and if renal biopsies are examined days or weeks after the initial episode, dilated tubules may be found lined by flat, regenerated epithelial cells. At first, patients with tubular necrosis show acute renal failure, but if they can be dialysed, a significant proportion recover reasonable renal function.

Renal Transplantation

This is an important development of recent years. Cases are selected so that histocompatibility differences are minimal; immunosuppression is always used to control rejection. Many renal grafts have now survived for several years. However, rejection is always liable to occur. The changes seen in the kidney following transplantation may be the result of ischaemia or they may be immunological. Some degree of ischaemic tubular necrosis is expected immediately following transplantation but this recovers. Cellular rejection becomes manifest by immunoblasts appearing in the peritubular capillaries, leading to vascular thrombosis and tubular necrosis. Humoral antibodies may cause an Arthus type of hypersensitivity giving acute arteritis. The kidney becomes swollen and pale with areas of haemorrhage and increasing necrosis. Renal damage may also develop as a result of the primary disease (hypertension, glomerulonephritis, etc.) affecting the transplant. There may also be a graft versus host reaction in the patient due to grafted lymphocytes escaping into the circulation.

Renal Tumours

Very small fibromas, leiomyomas and lipomas may be found in the subcapsular cortex but they are not of clinical significance. Tubular adenomas occur most frequently in scarred kidneys. They are usually tiny but if large they may be difficult to distinguish from cortical carcinomas. All tubular tumours over 3 cm diameter should be treated as malignant. A renal hamartoma (angiomyolipoma) may grow to a large size mimicking carcinoma. These are benign tumour-like malformations which may be found in patients with tuberose sclerosis.

Carcinoma of the Renal Parenchyma (*Hypernephroma*)

This accounts for three-quarters of all malignant tumours of the kidney and about 1 per cent of all malignant diseases. It characteristically consists of a spherical mass at one pole of the kidney and on section presents a mottled red, brown, yellow and grey surface, which is partly cystic. The different colours are due to haemorrhage, necrosis, fibrosis, and accumulation of fat in the tumour. The tumour may extend into the renal vein. Histologically, a tubular pattern is common, and frequently the tubular cells have a characteristic water-clear cytoplasm. An intracystic papillary pattern is another histological variant.

As might be expected from the tendency to extend down the renal vein, blood stream spread is common, and the lungs, brain, and bones are frequent sites for metastases. Lymph node metastases are found in about one-third of cases.

Tumours of the Renal Pelvis

These comprise about one-seventh of all renal tumours. Together with those of the ureter, their structure and behaviour are similar to those of the bladder, described below.

Wilms's Tumour

Wilms's tumour accounts for the remainder of primary malignant tumours and has been described on p. 120. It rarely occurs outside childhood and is most common in the first 5 years of life. The tumour is grey or white and infiltrates surrounding structures. Metastases are common both by way of lymphatics and blood stream.

Further Reading

Heptinstall, R. H. (1966) *Pathology of the Kidney*. London; Churchill.

The Urinary Bladder

Cystitis

Inflammation of the bladder mucosa or cystitis is common. It develops most frequently on the occasions when voiding of urine is inefficient. This occurs most commonly in men suffering from prostatic enlargement, and in women whose urethrae have become stretched and deformed as a result of parturition. Infection is also likely with neurogenic bladders and after catheterization or operations on the bladder. The mucous membrane is congested and oedematous and may become blackened, and encrusted with amorphous phosphates. The longer the inflammation persists, the more extensive will fibrosis of the underlying wall become. The epithelium dips into the underlying connective tissue and may form small cysts—*cystitis cystica*. Interstitial cystitis (*Hunner's ulcer*) occurs in middle-aged women but is of obscure aetiology. It may cause severe contraction of the bladder due to fibrous scarring.

Hypertrophy and Dilatation

The bladder is capable of considerable hypertrophy and dilatation if there is obstruction to urinary outflow in the urethra, as for example by prostatic enlargement. It is liable to become dilated if there is loss of nervous control. A hypertrophied but empty bladder has a thickened wall, with well-marked trabeculae on its inner surface. Sometimes obstruction to urinary outflow may lead to the formation of a diverticulum in the bladder wall which is liable to ulcerate and may perforate.

Tumours

The vast majority of bladder tumours are carcinomas or papillomas. They account for about 3 per cent of the deaths from all forms of malignant disease. The incidence of bladder carcinoma is greater in men than in women and it appears to be increasing. There is a recognized association with exposure to certain chemicals in industry. These include aniline dyes, benzidene, β-naphthylamine and 4-amino-diphenyl formerly used as an antioxidant in the rubber and plastics industry. Metabolites of trytophane are related to naphthylamine and this may account for some non-industrial carcinomas. There is a higher incidence in patients with schistosomiasis, but this may be the result of chronic inflammation of the bladder rather than a direct carcinogenic effect of the parasite. Squamous carcinoma is found in diverticula of the bladder. Congenital defect of the bladder and abdominal wall leaves the posterior surface of the bladder exposed (exstrophy) and this gives rise to chronic inflammation in which adenocarcinomas may develop.

Most tumours of the bladder recur and eventually infiltrate the underlying wall. Few are therefore 'benign' and the term *papilloma* is confined to about 5 per cent of papillary tumours in which the mucosa of the papillary folds is not heaped up or irregular and there is no invasion. *Carcinomas* are either papillary or solid in shape, the latter having a poor prognosis. Most are differentiated transitional cell carcinomas, but metaplasia is common and squamous carcinoma or adenocarcinoma are also found. Anaplastic carcinoma and adenocarcinoma may be difficult to distinguish from secondary carcinoma infiltrating the bladder. Primary carcinomas remain confined to the mucosa for some time but eventually infiltrate the muscle coat and perivesical tissues. Metastases to pelvic and paraaortic lymph nodes and by blood stream to liver and lungs occur late.

In children *embryonal rhabdomyosarcoma* may occur in the bladder. This is a rare tumour which is highly malignant and grows in a grape-like fashion into the lumen (botryoid sarcoma). The same type of tumour is found in the cervix and vagina of girls.

22 The Male Genital Tract

The Prostate

Benign Enlargement or Hyperplasia

Benign prostatic hyperplasia is a very common change in the prostate of ageing man. It is sometimes called myo-adenoma, but this is not an acceptable term, as the abnormality does not consist of a single nodule, but of an irregularly distributed overgrowth in the gland. Because of its limitation to the period of the male menopause, it is considered to result from the endocrine imbalance which occurs at that period of life.

When examined with the naked eye, the prostate may show considerable enlargement of much of the gland or the overgrowth may be limited to one part. The change does not affect the posterior portion of the gland. The lateral lobes of the anterior portion may be chiefly involved, but frequently a striking feature is a polypoid swelling of the middle portion which projects into the bladder cavity, exerting a flap valve effect on the flow of urine through the prostatic urethra. The swelling of the lateral lobes also stretches and kinks the urethra, so it is not surprising that the major complication of this disease is retention of urine. On section, ill defined vesicular or solid nodules are present in the fibrous stroma. Milky fluid exudes from the vesicles.

On histological examination, the nodules consist mainly of a great overgrowth of the prostatic glandular epithelium, the supporting fibromuscular tissue growing pari passu. The epithelial cells in some tubes become atrophic. Occasional nodules consist of smooth muscle and fibrous tissue only. Small infarcts sometimes develop, and there is variable chronic inflammation.

The chief complications of prostatic enlargement are acute or chronic retention of urine with or without superadded infection.

Carcinoma

Carcinoma accounts for 6 per cent of all tumour deaths in males. It affects the posterior lobes primarily so that the diagnosis is usually made by rectal examination. It has been shown that the carcinoma remains latent in the prostate gland in many people. Its frequency increases with age. The affected prostate is usually considerably indurated and on section is pale grey brown often with orange flecks because of its high fat content. It is an adenocarcinoma of very variable differentiation. It may spread into the rest of the gland to produce urinary obstruction or it may spread outwards, either by the regional lymphatics or the blood stream. It has a particular tendency to infiltrate widely into the bones, where the metastases are often osteosclerotic. A raised serum acid phosphatase is a common finding when such metastases are present. Oestrogens may cause involution of the carcinoma but the overall death rate is not greatly improved due to the increased incidence of coronary thrombosis with this therapy.

Inflammation

Acute prostatitis is rare. It usually develops as a result of infection in the bladder or posterior urethra or it may follow surgery and instrumentation. Chronic prostatitis leading to the formation of a hard shrunken prostate often containing a number of small calculi may be the result of gonoccal infection or it may be due to coliform organisms. Granulomatous prostatitis is seen in tuberculous infections. The prostate is affected in about three-quarters of the cases of genitourinary tuberculosis. Cavitating caseating granulomata may eventually destroy much of the gland. Non-specific granulomatous prostatitis produces a histological picture very similar to tuberculosis but acid-fast bacilli are not found. This reaction is caused by rupture of prostatic ducts often as a result of inflammation or obstruction due to benign hyperplasia. The released secretion initiates the tuberculoid granulomata. The gland becomes fibrotic and hard, and is frequently mistaken clinically for carcinoma.

Urethra and Penis

Acute urethritis may be due to gonococcal infection or it may be due to other veneral infections in which the organism is not identified. Reiter's syndrome—acute urethritis conjunctivitis and arthritis—appears to be due to a mycoplasmal infection. Gonococcal urethritis, in neglected cases may cause urethral stricture and it may lead to systemic disease resulting in suppurative arthritis, tenosynovitis and endocarditis. Urethral stricture may also be due to congenital stenosis, most commonly at the external meatus, or to trauma, including that following prostatectomy.

Penile infections include the veneral diseases. Primary *syphilis* develops as a chancre usually on the glans penis or prepuce, 2 to 6 weeks after exposure to infection. At first it is an indurated papule which breaks down to form a punched-out ulcer. The chronic inflammatory infiltrate contains many plasma cells and there is endarteritis of the small vessels around the ulcer. It heals to leave a fibrous scar. Secondary syphilis may involve the penis, scrotum and perianal skin causing warty growths (condylomata lata) in which spirochaetes are numerous. *Lymphogranuloma venereum* is a virus infection which leads to lymphatic obstruction due to granulomatous inflammation of inguinal and pelvic lymph nodes. The primary site of infection on the penis often escapes detection. The disease is more important in women, where the pelvic involvement causes fibrosis leading to rectal stricture. *Granuloma inguinale*, caused by the coccobacillus, *Donovania granulomatis*, rarely occurs in this country although it is endemic in the West Indies. The primary lesion on the penis is a spreading ulcer with surrounding chronic inflammation in which histiocytes containing the organism can be found. Involvement of inguinal lymph nodes causes sinuses and much scarring.

Tumours

Urethral tumours are rare. Transitional cell carcinoma may develop in the posterior urethra but in the penile urethra they are squamous carcinomas and occur near the meatus. Carcinoma of the penis is rare in this country but in parts of Africa and Asia it is one of the commonest forms of malignant disease. It presents on the glans or inner aspect of the prepuce as a fungating mass of squamous carcinoma. It metastasizes to inguinal lymph nodes. Premalignant dysplasia, similar to that in the cervix, may be seen in the penile skin before invasive carcinoma develops. Squamous carcinoma of the scrotum was known as 'chimney-sweeps' cancer' due to the carcinogenic effect of soot in this industry. It is still more common in town dwellers and in those working with tar.

The Testis

Miscellaneous Disorders

Cystic swellings are common in association with the testis. A *hydrocele* is due to the accumulation of fluid within the tunica vaginalis, the wall of which is usually thickened by fibrous tissue and may contain a few inflammatory cells. While some hydroceles may be a consequence of inflammation, the aetiology of most remains obscure. Cysts may also develop in association with the epididymis. These are lined by flattened epithelium and contain clear fluid in which spermatozoa may be identified, for which reason they are often called *spermatoceles*. The testis may become infected (*orchitis*). Mumps orchitis is a painful affliction complicating the parotitis in the adolescent or adult, and may cause infertility when there is bilateral testicular involvement. Acute bacterial orchitis is relatively rare but may follow prostatectomy. Tuberculosis may involve the testis by way of the blood stream or from the urinary tract. The infection usually starts in the epididymis and spreads from there into the testis itself later. In advanced cases the vas deferens and seminal vesicles may become infected. Gumma of the testis was an important differential diagnosis from malignant tumour in the days when tertiary syphilis was common. Syphilis can also cause a diffuse interstitial orchitis.

The spermatic cord may undergo spontaneous *torsion* resulting in venous infarction of the testis. Atrophy of the testes, whether due to primary testicular failure or as a result of pituitary failure, commonly results in sterility. Varying degrees of testicular atrophy are also associated with undescended testes in the adult and with the chromosomal abnormality of *Klinefelter's syndrome* (p. 99). In undescended testes there is atrophy of the germinal epithelium of the seminiferous tubules, thickening of the tubular basement membrane and often some degree of hypertrophy of the interstitial cells.

Tumours

Malignant tumours of the testis are rare accounting for 0·5 per cent of malignant tumours in men. Seminoma and teratoma, alone or in combination, account for about 85 per cent of these tumours. Malignant lymphoma arising in the testis accounts for a further 7 per cent of tumours. *Seminoma* occurs over a wide age range, but the maximum incidence is about 40. It is ten times more common in undescended testes, probably because of the increased frequency of dysgenetic gonads in this group. An identical tumour in females, dysgerminoma, is also more common in dysgenetic gonads associated with Turner's syndrome. Seminoma causes testicular swelling and on section is pearly grey. Histologically, it consists of sheets of spheroidal cells with pale vesicular nuclei together with foci of lymphocytes. It spreads early to the paraaortic lymph nodes near the renal vessels, and later by the blood stream to lungs and bone. It is extremely radiosensitive and has a good prognosis with 80 per cent 5-year survivals.

Teratomas of the testis are slightly less common than seminomas and have a peak age incidence about 30 years. Testicular teratomas, unlike those that arise in the ovary, are nearly all malignant. On section, the appearance of the tumour is variable but it is often cystic. The best differentiated (Teratoma Differentiated, TD) show no obvious malignant elements yet some metasatsize. No testicular teratoma is therefore diagnosed initially as benign. Less well differentiated tumours may show some malignant components mixed with differentiated tissues (Malignant Teratoma Intermediate Type A, MTIA), or all the tissues may appear malignant (Malignant Teratoma Intermediate Type B, MTIB, and Malignant Teratoma Anaplastic, MTA). Most testicular teratomas fall into the groups MTIA, MTIB. Malignant Teratoma Trophoblastic (MTT) is a highly malignant haemorrhagic tumour, containing syncytio- and cytotrophoblast similar to that in placental tumours. Gonadotrophin secreted by this tumour may cause a positive pregnancy test. Teratomas spread particularly by the blood stream to the lungs but may also involve paraaortic lymph nodes. They have a poor prognosis and are not sensitive to X-rays.

Malignant lymphoma occurs in the testis, apparently as a primary tumour. It is more likely to be bilateral than the other important testicular tumours and occurs later in life. Most of these tumours are highly malignant.

Tumours of the cord may cause scrotal swellings. These tumours are mainly derived from connective tissues and include fibromas, lipomas, leiomyomas and their malignant counterparts.

Further Reading

Collins, D. H. and Pugh, R. C. B. (1964) *The Pathology of Testicular Tumours*. Edinburgh, Livingstone.

23 The Female Genital Tract

The Vulva

Pruritus vulvae is a frequent complaint which in many instances has no organic basis. It is associated with two conditions which frequently are indistinguishable clinically, one of which shows a distinct tendency to progress to squamous cell carcinoma. They are lichen sclerosis et atrophicus and leukoplakia vulvae.

Lichen sclerosis is an atrophic change in the skin which may develop anywhere on the body. It is, however, of importance in the vulva because it may progress to leukoplakia. The epidermis, histologically, appears atrophic with flattening of papillae and the outer part of the dermis is very oedematous.

Leukoplakia vulvae consists macroscopically of a thickening and whitening of the skin. Histologically, the skin is hyperplastic and the epidermal papillae project irregularly into the underlying dermis. In the later stages of the disease, the normal polarity of the squamous epithelium also becomes lost, and the individual cells vary in size and may show increased mitotic activity. The underlying dermis shows chronic inflammation and eventually becomes sclerotic. The development of squamous cell carcinoma is a definite risk but is by no means inevitable.

Carcinoma of the vulva accounts for a little less than 5 per cent of cancers of the female genital tract. Its behaviour is similar to that of squamous cell carcinoma elsewhere in the skin, with a tendency to metastasize to the lymph nodes of the groin.

Bartholin's cyst occurs in the posterior part of the labia minora. It results from duct obstruction following acute or recurrent inflammation, often caused by gonococci. The cyst is lined by cubical or columnar cells of the duct and may contain acini of the gland in its wall.

The Cervix Uteri

Cervicitis

Acute cervicitis may be a feature of gonorrhoea. Chronic cervicitis is an extremely common condition that is frequently the result of trauma causing ectropion of the external os or of a cervical erosion. A cervical erosion is produced by glandular endocervical epithelium extending on to the pars vaginalis of the cervix where it invariably becomes infected, producing abundant mucus and a vaginal discharge. The cause of the erosion appears to be linked with an hormonal imbalance. The times of life when it is found most frequently are at birth (from the high maternal steroid level), at puberty, with oral contraceptive therapy and during pregnancy. An erosion has a velvety appearance and tends to bleed easily. Microscopically the following features are usually found: (1) chronic inflammatory cell infiltration, (2) a cluster of minute polyps of chronic inflammatory granulation tissue, partially covered by cubical epithelium, (3) cystic dilatation of the submucous glands (the cysts seen naked eye), and (4) squamous metaplasia of the columnar epithelium. The last can sometimes appear so atypical that discrimination is needed to distinguish it from carcinoma-in-situ (see below).

Mucous polyp is a common overgrowth arising within the cervical canal and having the same basic structure. It is liable to ulcerate and bleed.

Carcinoma

Carcinoma of the cervix uteri is one of the commoner causes of death from malignant disease in women, accounting for approximately 5 per cent, but being less frequent than the digestive tract, breast, bronchus and ovary. A great deal of interest is being taken at the present time in the use of exfoliative cytology in the early diagnosis of this disease. In gynaecological clinics, routine examination of cervical smears from patients without obvious cancer reveals slightly less than 1 per cent of cases with exfoliated cells having the characters of malignant disease. Cervical biopsy has indicated that the majority of these have carcinoma-in-situ, i.e. carcinoma limited to the lining epithelium; a few have early invasive cancer. Some cases of carcinoma-in-situ have been followed up without treatment and it appears that at least 25 per cent will progress within a few years to invasive carcinoma. It is possible, therefore, that the incidence of carcinoma of the cervix could be much reduced by the widespread and systematic use of exfoliative cytology.

Carcinoma of the cervix is unusual below 30. Two-thirds of the patients are between 40 and 60 years of age. There is a definite association with sexual intercourse being commonest in those having intercourse young and frequently. It is commoner in the lower socio-economic groups. It usually arises at or near the external os. Macroscopically the tumour is nodular, ulcerated, and tends to bleed easily. It will have infiltrated the whole of the cervical stroma and vaginal vault in a high proportion of cases when first seen. Histologically, 95 per cent of cases are of squamous cell structure, the relatively rare adenocarcinomas arising always within the canal. The squamous tumours are frequently rather poorly differentiated. Carcinoma of the cervix tends to spread early by local infiltration of the parametrium so that the lateral wall of the pelvis eventually becomes implicated, with obstruction of the ureters. The bladder, rectum, and peritoneum may be penetrated. Spread to pelvic lymph nodes is also common.

The Body of the Uterus

Uterine Curettings

Gynaecological specimens make up about half of all those handled by a routine surgical histological laboratory, and a large proportion of them consist of curettings from the endometrium. The chief reasons for the submission of curettings are as follows: (1) the diagnosis and treatment of incomplete abortion through the identification of decidua of pregnancy and of chorionic villi, (2) the diagnosis of carcinoma of the uterine body, (3) the diagnosis of cystic glandular hyperplasia, an index of functional bleeding, (4) the establishment that ovulation has occurred, as part of the examination for infertility, by the demonstration that the endometrium is in the secretory phase, and (5) the diagnosis of genital tuberculosis, by the demonstration of endometrial tubercles in premenstrual curettings.

Curettings reveal the phase of the menstrual cycle with considerable precision. During the first five days of the cycle the endometrium breaks down so that only the basal glands remain. These regenerate surface epithelium and from then until the fourteenth day the glands and stroma proliferate under the influence of oestrogen. Mitoses are numerous, producing elongation of the glands. At ovulation and under the influence of progesterone, subnuclear vacuoles appear in the glandular epithelium; these vacuoles pass to the luminal side of the cell by the nineteenth day. From the twentieth day secretion appears in the gland lumen. Stromal cells develop more cytoplasm and the stroma becomes compact. From the twenty-fifth day polymorph leucocytes infiltrate the stroma. In the premenstrual endometrium blood leaks into the stroma and this is followed by constriction of the spiral arteries and breakdown of the endometrium.

Cystic Glandular Hyperplasia

This hyperplasia of the endometrium occurs with anovulatory menstrual cycles especially at the menopause. It gives rise to irregular bleeding referred to as metropathia haemorrhagica. Prolonged oestrogen stimulation causes excessive endometrial proliferation resulting in a thickened spongy endometrium. Histologically the glands are cystic and lined by stratified epithelium. With fluctuation in the oestrogen level, pseudomenstrual breakdown occurs, often accompanied by heavy bleeding resulting in iron deficiency anaemia. An abnormal response in the endometrium may result in focal proliferation of non-secretory cystic glandular hyperplasia resulting in an endometrial polyp. At the menopause, gradual fall in oestrogen activity results in involution of the hyperplasia but the glands remain cystic—senile cystic endometrium.

Leiomyoma (Fibroid) of Myometrium

Approximately one-tenth of all patients in gynaecological practice suffer from fibroids. The tumour shows a wide range of presentations. It may be single or multiple and numbering up to one hundred. It may be of pinhead size, or be so large as to cause massive distortion of the uterus. Most leiomyomas occupy an intramural position, but some exist as either subserous or submucous polyps, projecting from the peritoneal surface or into the endometrial cavity respectively. Occasionally the tumour will form in the cervical myometrium or extra-mural in the broad ligament. Leiomyomas are usually hard and difficult to cut. Their fasciculated pale grey cut surface has been likened to watered silk. They are prone to degenerative changes, among which necrosis, oedema, haemorrhage, cyst formation and calcification are observable macroscopically. Haemorrhagic necrosis is liable to develop in the pregnant uterus and in those on oral contraceptives (red degeneration). Occasionally the myoma may become completely impregnated with calcium (a 'womb stone'). The histological picture consists of interweaving bundles of smooth muscle fibres in a varying amount of fibrous stroma, which contains a number of medium-sized vascular channels, and frequently undergoes hyaline 'degeneration'. Although the tumour can usually be shelled out from the surrounding myometrium, the line of separation may not be clear cut histologically. The aetiology of these tumours is still obscure. The fact that they are limited to the reproductive era indicates that they are endocrine-dependent. Structurally they are similar to the vascular leiomyomas that sometimes develop in the skin. Occasionally leimyosarcomatous change develops.

Decidual Cast

During pregnancy progestational stimulation of the endometrium results in secretory hyperplasia. The glands become excessively tortuous, the epithelium pale and vacuolated and the nuclei protrude into the lumen. These changes are known as the Arias-Stella phenomenon. The stromal cells acquire abundant cytoplasm to form decidua. If there is a uterine pregnancy, chorionic villi become embedded in this decidua. However, if there is an ectopic (tubal) pregnancy (p. 244) the endometrial changes occur without chorionic villi. Death of the foetus may be followed by shedding of the endometrium as a decidual cast. Excessive decidua may also accompany prolonged progestagen therapy. If there is no oestrogen priming of the glands these remain atrophic so that the glands and stroma become 'out of step'. Withdrawal of progestagen may result in a decidual cast being shed.

Endometritis

Chronic inflammation of the endometrium commonly follows abortion; it may be the result of chronic gonococcal infection also affecting the fallopian tubes or it may be due to tuberculosis. Tuberculous granulomata take some weeks to develop so that they are not seen in the post-menstrual or proliferative phase of the menstrual cycle. If tuberculosis is suspected, curettage is best postponed until the premenstrual phase of the cycle. Endometrial tuberculosis is always secondary to tuberculosis elsewhere in the body particularly in the urinary tract and lungs. Endometritis may occur in older women as a result of endometrial carcinoma.

Carcinoma of the Endometrium

Carcinoma of the body of the uterus is becoming more common, the death rate now being about half that of carcinoma of the cervix. It occurs particularly in nulliparous women at the time of the menopause or later. In some cases it is seen to arise in cystic glandular hyperplasia and is associated with excess oestrogen which may be derived from oestrogen-secreting ovarian tumours such as thecomas and granulosa cell tumours (p. 247). It is commoner in obese diabetic patients.

The tumour projects into the uterine cavity as a papillary mass. Myometrial invasion is often limited to the superficial layers. Tumour may extend into the endocervix and into the submucosal lymphatics in the upper third of the vagina. Most of the tumours are well differentiated adenocarcinomas but squamous metaplasia may occur to form an adenoacanthoma. Metastasis to the ovaries is common, but the tumour rarely becomes widespread outside the pelvis. The prognosis is considerably more favourable than for carcinoma of the cervix.

Endometrial Sarcoma

The endometrial stroma may become malignant producing sheets of undifferentiated cells or there may be differentiation into a variety of mesodermal tissues, including glandular epithelium, to form a mixed mesodermal tumour (p. 120). Endometrial sarcomas are considerably more malignant than the more common carcinomas and there is often infiltration through the myometrium into the parametrial tissues at the time of clinical presentation.

Adenomyosis

In this condition the myometrium usually shows an asymmetric swelling without clear boundaries, the cut surface of which is similar to normal myometrium except that small cystic spaces may be present, which are sometimes blood-stained. Histologically these cystic spaces are seen to be due to islands of endometrium in the myometrium, the endometrial tubules usually appearing hyperplastic and of non-secretory type. The condition is considered to arise as a result of penetration of the endometrium into the underlying myometrium.

The Uterine (Fallopian) Tubes

Inflammation

Acute and chronic inflammation may result from inflammation elsewhere in the genital tract. Examples are puerperal sepsis, gonorrhoea, and non-specific cervicitis. Tuberculous salpingitis is now a relatively uncommon disease within the female genital tract. All these inflammatory lesions give an obstructive basis for infertility. The inflammation may lead to accumulation of pus within the lumen (pyosalpinx), or extend to involve the ovary (tubovarian abscess). It may settle to leave a distended tube containing watery fluid (hydrosalpinx).

Ectopic Pregnancy

Usually because of the development of previous inflammatory changes in the uterine tube, the progress of a fertilized ovum may become arrested in the tube, leading to an ectopic pregnancy. The pregnancy terminates spontaneously in the early stages, as a consequence of the haemorrhage which results from the trophoblastic activity in this abnormal situation. The lesion is an important cause of an acute abdominal emergency in women. The endometrial changes have been described on page 242.

Tumours

The uterine tubes are a very uncommon site for primary tumours. They are, however, more frequently involved in extensions of carcinoma from the uterine body or ovaries.

The Ovaries

Cysts are prone to develop in the ovaries. For convenience they can be divided into non-neoplastic and neoplastic cysts.

Non-neoplastic Cysts

(a) *Germinal inclusion cysts.* These are usually small, not visible to the naked eye and are lined by a single layer of cuboidal or columnar cells. (b) *Follicular cysts.* These are the commonest cysts to be observed in the ovary, are unilocular, differ from developing follicles in being over 2·5 cm in diameter, and are filled with clear fluid rich in oestrogen. There may be associated non-secretory hyperplasia of the endometrium due to prolonged oestrogen stimulation. Histologically, the cysts are seen to be lined by granulosa and theca interna cells. They may be particularly numerous and prominent in the Stein-Leventhal syndrome in which the combination of amenorrhoea and hirsutism exists. (c) *Corpus luteum cysts.* These result when there is an aberration of the normal regression of the corpora lutea. The cyst fluid may be clear or consist of blood. (d) *Endometrial cysts.* Ectopic endometrium may be found in the ovary, forming the wall of a cyst. The endometrium is rarely fully developed; the commonest arrangement seen histologically is cuboidal or columnar epithelium lining the cyst with well-developed endometrial stroma, beneath which there may be clusters of siderocytes indicative of previous haemorrhage. The cyst lumen often contains blood. The likely causes of 'chocolate cysts' of ovary are thus haemorrhagic corpus luteum and endometrial cyst.

Parovarian cysts are derived from embryonic Mullerian and Wolffian duct remnants in the hilum of the ovary and lateral end of the fallopian tube. They are simple cysts lined by cubical or flattened epithelium.

Neoplastic Cysts

(a) *Mucinous cystadenoma.* This accounts for 25 per cent of all ovarian tumours, and is the one which produces the biggest forms. The outer surface is smooth and the cut surface is multilocular with thin walls. The cavities are filled with clear mucin. Histologically the cyst walls are lined by tall columnar epithelium, with basal nuclei and pale cytoplasm because of the contained mucin. Rupture of these cysts, as with similar cystic tumours in the pancreas and appendix, may result in seeding of tumour cells throughout the peritoneal cavity. They continue to produce mucin and give rise to pseudomyxoma (myxoma) peritonei. (b) *Serous cystadenoma.* This also accounts for 25 per cent of all ovarian tumours. About 20 per cent are bilateral. The outer surface may be smooth or show fine warty outgrowths. It is commonly unilocular and filled with clear fluid.

The inner lining may be smooth or covered with warty ingrowths which are found more frequently than the outgrowths already mentioned. Microscopically it is seen to be lined by a single layer of flattened epithelium, the warty structures having fibrous cores. Malignant change occurs more frequently than with the mucinous variety. (c) *Dermoid cyst*. This accounts for 10 per cent of ovarian tumours. It is liable to be smaller than the cystadenomas. The lumen is often filled with pale greasy material which may contain abundant hairs. A ridge of tissue projects a little into the lumen at one point on the circumference, in which a tooth or bony structures may be obvious. The histological picture, particularly in this region, shows the lining to be of hair-bearing skin under which may be found a wide variety of tissues consisting of normal-looking cells, but not showing the relationship commonly observed in the normal body. Malignant change in ovarian dermoid tumours is very rare.

Carcinoma of the Ovary

Carcinoma of the ovary accounts for approximately 6 per cent of all female deaths from malignant disease, being slightly more frequent than carcinoma of the cervix. It may be primary or metastatic. *Primary carcinoma* may be either predominantly cystic or mainly solid, the relative frequency being approximately in the ratio of 4:1. The cystic forms originate in the corresponding cystadenomas and are either serous or mucinous cystadenocarcinomas, the former being much the more common. Features of malignancy in these tumours include solid areas in a cystic tumour, necrosis, infiltration of the capsule and pelvic adhesions. Histologically there is heaping-up of the lining epithelium with nuclear pleomorphism and mitotic activity. The solid carcinomas are adenocarcinomas which vary in differentiation from case to case. Spread of all forms is usually first to the peritoneum and omentum, so that ascites and adhesions between bowel loops frequently develop. Spread may also take place into the rest of the genital tract, and metastases in the endometrium are common. Pelvic and paraaortic lymph nodes are frequently involved but haematogenous spread is less usual. The 5-year survival is approximately 15 to 20 per cent. Metastases to the pleural cavity may give rise to a malignant effusion. *Secondary carcinoma*. The ovaries are quite frequently the seat of secondary carcinoma, the commonest primary sites being the alimentary tract, especially the stomach

(Krukenberg tumours), the uterine body and breast. Krukenberg tumours may mimic primary ovarian fibromas although histologically the mucin-secreting carcinoma cells reveal their true identity. It seems probable that gastric carcinomas invade the ovaries by transperitoneal spread, although in other cases lymphatic and haematogenous spread may be more important.

Functional Tumours of the Ovary

Some tumours of the ovary produce hormones, mainly oestrogen. The most important of these tumours is derived from, and histologically resembles, the granulosal cells of the developing follicle—the *granulosa cell tumour*. A closely related tumour is the *thecoma*. Both of these tumours are well circumscribed and on section may appear yellow. Granulosa cell tumours often contain cysts or areas of haemorrhage, whereas thecomas more frequently resemble fibromas. Both types of tumour are usually benign in their behaviour although 30 per cent recur after excision. The effects of the high oestrogen output is to cause endometrial hyperplasia or carcinoma, leiomyomata of the myometrium and cystic hyperplasia of the breast. Masculinizing effects are produced by the *arrhenoblastoma*, a tumour of varying histological pattern but often containing tubular structures and cells resembling the interstitial cells of the testis. About 20 per cent of the tumours recur and metastasize. In addition to these functional tumours, it is now clear that many types of ovarian tumour occasionally may be associated with excess oestrogen production.

Other Ovarian Tumours

Brenner tumours are benign fibrous tumours which contain islands of squamous epithelium possibly derived from islands of metaplastic surface epithelium commonly found on the fallopian tube and ovary —Walthard's nests. These tumours may occur in the wall of mucinous cystadenomas.

Fibromas are common and are derived from the stroma of the ovarian cortex. The surface epithelium may be invaginated into the fibroma to form an adenofibroma or cystadenofibroma. Some fibromas represent the end stages of thecomas or Brenner tumours and careful search may be required to identify their true nature.

Dysgerminoma, a rare tumour identical to the seminoma of the testis, arises more commonly in dysgenetic gonads, e.g. Turner's syndrome. They metastasize to paraaortic lymph nodes and by the blood stream.

Torsion of the Ovary

Torsion of the ovary is usually secondary to an ovarian neoplasm. Those most likely to undergo torsion are heavy, benign tumours on a long pedicle such as dermoid cysts and fibromas. Malignant tumours rarely undergo torsion because of pelvic adhesions. Torsion results in venous occlusion, oedema and infarction of the ovary and attached fallopian tube.

Endometriosis

The presence of ectopic endometrium in the ovary has already been mentioned. It may be found in the uterine tube, on the outside of the uterus, on the pelvic peritoneum, the bowel, the bladder and even the umbilicus, as well as in less frequent sites. Multiple lesions are usual. Macroscopically, the foci of endometriosis are small usually puckered scars, which contain tar-like blood-stained fluid. Microscopically, the combination of endometrial epithelium and stroma is diagnostic, and tissue reaction to shed blood is usually present. The pathogenesis of this condition is obscure. It may be due to growth of particles of endometrium transported from the uterus through the uterine tube or by metaplastic transformation of tissues having the factor in common that they are derived from primitive coelom. As neither explanation can account for all cases, it is possible that more than one factor is involved in the formation of these lesions.

Tumours of the Placenta

Two tumours are derived from the trophoblastic covering of the chorionic villi of the placenta. These are *hydatidiform mole* and *chorioncarcinoma*. There is a moderate degree of trophoblastic proliferation in hydatidiform mole, the chorionic villi become hydropic and avascular, resembling small grapes. These are usually benign but may progress to chorioncarcinoma. In the latter, the trophoblastic proliferation is considerable and it is usually impossible to recognize any villous structure. Chorioncarcinoma is a highly malignant and invasive tumour, which often appears haemorrhagic. Both tumours are associated with the secretion of large quantities of *chorionic gonadotrophin* which may give strong-positive pregnancy tests. They also cause the formation of ovarian cysts lined by luteinized theca cells—*theca lutein cysts*.

Pre-eclamptic Toxaemia of Pregnancy

This disease occurs usually in late pregnancy. It is characterized by hypertension, proteinuria and oedema. More severe cases have fits and are referred to as eclampsia. The placenta undergoes premature ageing causing foetal distress. In eclampsia, there is swelling of endothelial cells and thickening of basement membranes in renal glomeruli. The liver may show periportal necrosis which may progress to massive necrosis. The cause of these changes is not clearly known but appears to be related to a placental factor for there is often dramatic improvement following the termination of pregnancy.

Further Reading

Haines, M. and Taylor, C. W. (1962) *Gynaecological Pathology*. London, Churchill

Novak, E. R. and Woodruff, J. D. (1967) *Novak's Gynaecologic and Obstretic Pathology*. 6th edn. Philadelphia, Saunders

24 The Breast

Cystic Hyperplasia

(Adenosis; Chronic Cystic Mastitis)

This change is extremely common in female breasts during the reproductive period, producing an ill-defined lumpiness of the breast tissue. Sometimes one of the lumps may be more prominent than the remainder and require examination by operation to exclude the possibility that carcinoma has developed. The cut surface of an affected breast shows the presence of poorly defined nodules of rubbery pale grey tissue studded with cysts of varying size. A single large cyst is commonly the basis of the lump operated on to exclude carcinoma. The cysts may contain clear or thick brownish fluid. Histologically, the important features include: (1) proliferation of breast ductules and lobules—*adenosis*, (2) sclerosis of the intralobular connective tissue, (3) cystic dilatation of ductules with retention of secretion and surrounding chronic inflammation, (4) metaplasia of the lining cubical epithelium to resemble apocrine epithelium, (5) infolding of the lining epithelium—*papillomatosis* and (6) proliferation of the lining epithelium of ductules and ducts—*epitheliosis*. It is this epitheliosis which causes much concern, for transitions can be traced between it and intraduct carcinoma. In addition there is statistical evidence to show that carcinoma of the breast is four to five times more frequent in breasts which are already affected by cystic hyerplasia. Occasionally breasts show severe adenosis and a reactive fibroblast proliferation—*sclerosing adenosis*, which may mimic carcinoma clinically and histologically. This is not primarily an inflammatory disease and the term 'mastitis' is therefore unfortunate. It appears to be due to an hormonal imbalance, particularly an excess of oestrogen over progesterone.

Duct Ectasia

The ducts become blocked by creamy material and there is often rupture of the ducts causing an inflammatory reaction in which foamy histiocytes predominate. The fibrous scarring may produce a clinical lump in the breast.

Fat Necrosis

Following injury, fat released by ruptured fat cells is taken up by macrophages. There is an accompanying chronic inflammatory reaction with resultant scarring. This results in a local lump in the breast which may be mistaken for carcinoma.

Breast Abscess

This is usually found in the lactating breast. Infection often gains access to the breast tissue through a crack in the nipple. The changes in the breast are those of acute inflammation.

Galactocele

This also occurs in a lactating breast. It is a cyst formed by duct obstruction and contains milk. There is a risk of infection if untreated.

Fibro-adenoma

Fibro-adenoma is a common tumour, which is not often more than about 3 cm. in diameter. It is pearly grey to the naked eye and has a distinct line of cleavage from the surrounding breast. Its cut surface contains small clefts and pits. Histologically the commonest picture is one of stretched epithelium lining slit-like lumens and being distorted by irregular overgrowth of the characteristically loose mucoid fibrous stroma (the intracanalicular form). Less commonly the tubules are small and circular, and separated from each other by evenly disposed fibrous tissue (the pericanalicular form). The tumours tend to regress with age, and may become hyaline, calcified or ossified. Occasionally, especially if they grow to a large size, low grade sarcomatous change develops in the stroma (Brodie's tumour or cystosarcoma phylloides).

Duct Papilloma

Duct papilloma occurs as a small solitary tumour, usually in a main duct near a nipple, or as a multiple phenomenon with wide distribution deeper in the breast. In the latter case, they are usually found in a cystic and hyperplastic breast. Most of the lesions remain benign: some undergo carcinomatous transformation. They commonly present with bleeding from the nipple.

Carcinoma of the Breast

Carcinoma of the breast is the commonest cause of death due to malignant disease among women, accounting for approximately 20 per cent of the total. The alimentary tract taken altogether accounts for more deaths (32 per cent), but the individual organs are less frequently involved than the breast; for example, the stomach 12 per cent, and the large bowel 17 per cent. About one in every 20 women in this country will eventually develop a carcinoma of breast. The tumour occasionally develops in males. Most cases are found between the ages of 40 and 60 years. The disease is more likely to be found in those patients who have had either absence or disturbance of normal mammary function. For example it is more common in single women than married ones, and more common in those married women who are subfertile, have a high miscarriage and stillbirth rate, and errors of lactation. The upper and outer quadrant of the breast is the most frequent site affected, with the centre and upper inner quadrant next in order, the lower segments being the least often involved. Small infiltrating tumours are often peripheral, whereas the larger variants tend to be more central, especially in older people. The macroscopic and microscopic pictures vary widely. The commonest form is a very hard (scirrhous) nodule, whose cut surface averages about one centimetre square and which sends short processes into the adjacent breast tissue. The tumour usually presents a concave grey cut surface, often bearing creamy flecks. A larger and softer (encephaloid) form often shows a surrounding lymphocytic infiltrate which may indicate a host cellular immune response to the tumour. These cases have a more favourable prognosis than those with scirrhous tumours. Mucoid (colloid) carcinoma occurs in older women and also has a more favourable prognosis. The mucoid appearance is due to abundant mucus secretion by tumour cells. Papillary carcinomas have already been mentioned. These may be cured by excision before there is extensive invasion of the stalk. During lactation, a rapidly growing carcinoma may give the clinical appearance of acute inflammation. These tumours, fortunately rare, have a very poor prognosis. Tumour infiltration may make it difficult to move the overlying skin freely, and through lymphatic obstruction may make the latter oedematous (*peau d'orange*). Nipple retraction is quite common and, in neglected cases, the skin may become ulcerated. The tumour may also, in the later stages, become attached to the chest wall. The commonest histological picture is that of solid alveoli and trabeculae of undifferentiated carcinoma. In some of the remaining cases tubule formation may be quite conspicuous. The fibrous stromal reaction varies considerably. Clumps of tumour cells are frequently conspicuous within the lymphatic channels. Malignant proliferation may be confined to the larger ducts obstructing their lumen. These *intraduct carcinomas* are cured by local excision as they do not metastasize until they invade.

Spread

Extension beyond the confines of the breast is frequent. Indeed, surgeons consider that well over half of their cases of breast carcinoma are incurable at the time of operation. The regional lymph nodes frequently contain metastases and, since most tumours are in the upper and outer quadrant, the axillary lymph nodes are commonly implicated later also involving supraclavicular nodes. However, the inaccessible internal mammary chain of lymphatics are infiltrated in a high proportion of all cases, so that intrathoracic spread is likely. Blood-borne metastases are most frequently found in the lung, liver, brain and bones. The bone involvement may be localized, causing a pathological fracture, or widespread through most of the bones leading to diminished haemopoiesis. The bony metastases may be predominantly osteosclerotic.

Among the many varied presentations of carcinoma of the breast, one is of special interest—*Paget's disease* of the nipple. Here the nipple shows an eczematous change which on section, is seen to be associated with the presence of large pale-staining cells in the epidermis. A high proportion of patients with Paget's disease of the nipple will develop carcinoma in the underlying breast, usually arising in the atypically hyperplastic ducts which are commonly a feature in these patients. The nature of the Paget's cells is still a matter of debate. The fact that they may rarely occur without underlying carcinoma indicates that they are not secondary tumour infiltration of the epidermis. They may represent a form of primary intraepidermal carcinoma induced by carcinogenic secretion in breast ducts. This would account for the association with breast carcinoma.

25 The Thyroid, Parathyroids, Adrenals and Pituitary

The Thyroid Gland

Goitres

These are enlarged thyroid glands. They may be nodular or diffuse.

The pituitary stimulates the thyroid through the action of thyroid stimulating hormone (TSH) causing proliferation and increased activity of the thyroid epithelium. In the presence of adequate iodine supplies this causes an increased output of thyroxine into the blood, which suppresses further pituitary output of TSH. In the absence of adequate iodine supplies, as in mountainous areas or following therapy with goitrogenic substances, the output of thyroxine fails, and the prolonged TSH stimulation of the thyroid causes a *simple goitre*. As expected, the gland is fleshy and cellular with little colloid stored in it. When the demand for thyroxine diminishes or when iodine supplies are restored, the gland undergoes involution with accumulation of large quantities of pale-staining colloid to form a *colloid goitre*. This may be *diffuse* or, with recurrent stimulation and involution, it may become *nodular*. In these nodular goitres, haemorrhage is very likely to occur and results in focal scars. *Toxic goitres* are associated with the increased output of thyroxine either due to an independently functioning nodule or due to stimulation by long-acting thyroid stimulator (see p. 256). This thyroid overactivity results in thyrotoxicosis or hyperthyroidism. Other causes of goitre are carcinoma and thyroiditis including Hashimoto's disease.

Hyperthyroidism

This disease occurs in two main forms, *exophthalmic goitre* (primary thyrotoxicosis or Graves' disease) and *toxic nodular goitre* (secondary thyrotoxicosis). Graves' disease is associated with the presence in the serum of long-acting thyroid stimulator (LATS) which has an effect on the thyroid gland similar to but more prolonged than that of TSH. However LATS is not produced by the pituitary and is not suppressed by increased output of thyroxine. It has the properties of a γ-globulin and is believed to be an autoantibody. These patients may have other thyroid antibodies in their serum similar to those found in Hashimoto's disease and some patients with Graves' disease progress to Hashimoto's disease. Graves' disease affects particularly young and middle-aged adults, being much commoner in women. There is exophthalmos and evidence of increased metabolic activity. Some muscle weakness and wasting are common but a fully-developed myopathy is rare. Cardiac arrythmia occurs in older patients. Pretibial myxoedema may develop and is due to the accumulation of mucopolysaccharides in the dermis. The diffusely involved gland is very vascular and firmer than normal. It feels tough on section, the cut surface is fleshy, and colloid is hard to identify. Microscopically, the follicles are hyperplastic, being lined by columnar epithelium thrown up into papillary infoldings. Colloid is scanty and pale staining with peripheral vacuolation where it lies adjacent to follicular cells. Lymphoid follicles with germinal centres are scattered through the gland. Apart from the lymphoid tissue, thought to be a manifestation of autoimmunity, the hyperplastic appearance is not pathognomonic of Graves' disease for it may be due to TSH stimulation and is found in patients treated with carbimazole which prevents the formation of iodotyrosine and thyroxine thus stimulating pituitary activity by 'negative feedback'. The histological picture of Graves' disease is usually obscured in the surgically excised gland because pre-operative iodine therapy makes the thyroid gland revert in the direction of normal.

Toxic nodules produce excessive quantities of thyroid hormone but it is not associated with high levels of LATS in their serum. Secondary hyperthyroidism occurs in older patients and the overactivity is more likely to be associated with cardiac arrythmia; exophthalmos is not a feature. Thyrotoxicosis should always be considered in the diagnosis of unexplained cardiac arrythmia in elderly patients. Radioactive iodine uptake by the gland reveals that it is concentrated in the 'hot nodule'.

Macroscopically and histologically the nodule shows the features of hyerplasia but the remainder of the gland shows no clear-cut differences from non-toxic nodular goitre. The reason for a single nodule showing increased function is not yet clear but the fact that the normal gland shows focal uptake of radioactive iodine may provide part of the explanation.

Thyroiditis

Acute thyroiditis may complicate a local inflammatory reaction such as a carbuncle in the neck or it may be a complication of septicaemia. *Subacute, giant-cell, thyroiditis* (de Quervain's disease) is an inflammatory lesion which presents as a diffuse, tender enlargement of the gland. It is probably of viral origin and cases occur in association with mumps. Histologically, giant cell—histiocyte granulomata, similar to those found in sarcoid, occur in thyroid follicles and ingest colloid resulting in focal scarring; myxoedema is uncommon. *Hashimoto's disease* (struma lymphomatosa) is an autoimmune form of thyroiditis. It occurs particularly in middle-aged women as a firm, diffuse enlargement of the thyroid gland leading to loss of function and myxoedema. The serum can be shown by precipitating, tanned red cell agglutination, complement fixing and immunofluorescence antibody techniques to contain antibodies to thyroglobulin and various components of thyroid cytoplasm. Many of these patients also have antibodies in their serum which react with gastric parietal cells and may be associated with megaloblastic anaemia due to absence of intrinsic factor (p. 182). Macroscopically the gland shows uniform enlargement but remains confined by the capsule. The cut surface is pale. Histologically there is infiltration by lymphocytes and plasma cells destroying the normal follicular pattern. Colloid is scanty; epithelial cells are aggregated in small foci and show metaplasia to large eosinophilic cells—Askanazy cells. Fibrous tissue gradually replaces the cellular infiltrate and destroyed follicles. *Focal lymphocytic thyroiditis* is found in hyperplastic glands of primary thyrotoxicosis. When this thyroiditis is extensive and associated with the formation of germinal centres, there is a tendency for patients to develop myxoedema. It is, therefore, a feature of some importance in thyroidectomy specimens. It shows many features in common with Hashimoto's disease. *Riedel's thyroiditis* is a rare form of thyroiditis in which there is fibrous replacement of the gland with involvement of surrounding tissues causing tracheal or oesophageal obstruction. It is usually mistaken clinically for carcinoma. The aetiology of the disease is not known. In spite of extensive destruction of the gland, myxoedema is seen in only a minority of cases.

Hypothyroidism

In children this may be the result of congenital absence of the thyroid gland or failure of one of the enzyme systems in the gland necessary for the formation of thyroxine (dyshormonogenetic goitre). It may be due to iodine deficiency during intrauterine life. In adults Hashimoto's disease is one of the most important causes of hypothyroidism. Primary atrophy (chronic atrophic thyroiditis) may develop in adult life, the histological picture being that of fibrous replacement of follicles but lymphocytic infiltration is usually slight. Antithyroid drugs, thyroidectomy, irradiation and pituitary failure may all cause loss of thyroid function. The result is the clinical picture of *cretinism* in infants and *myxoedema* in adults. A cretin shows failure of mental and physical development. The skin is cold, dry and puffy. The tongue is large and protrudes. Myxoedema in adults may be inapparent until it has reached an advanced stage. The puffiness of the skin is caused by infiltration of the dermis by mucopolysaccharides. The skin is cold, the hair brittle, scanty and dry. There is hoarseness due to swelling of the vocal cords. Hyperlipidaemia leads to coronary ischaemia but this may be less obvious clinically in untreated cases due to bradycardia and low cardiac output. Impairment of mental function may result in psychoses or coma.

Tumours

Adenoma

The distinction between adenoma and the nodules of a nodular goitre is not clear. The term adenoma is usually reserved for a nodule which is well circumscribed, surrounded by a fibrous capsule, compressing the adjacent thyroid tissue and having a histological pattern different from the rest of the gland. An adenoma is usually fleshy and histologically the follicles may resemble immature (foetal adenoma) or mature (follicular adenoma) thyroid. These tumours are prone to haemorrhage and cystic degeneration. Haemorrhage into a retrosternal adenoma may cause sudden and severe obstruction of the thoracic inlet. Very few adenomata have been shown to undergo malignant change.

Carcinoma

This is a relatively rare cause of death from malignant disease but it is important in that it often affects young adults and the metastases may be suitable for treatment with radioactive iodine. Previous X-ray therapy of the thyroid gland increases the risk of developing carcinoma but there is usually a latent period of 10 years or more before the tumour develops. The likelihood of radioiodine therapy leading to the development of carcinoma has still to be evaluated, but this potential risk should be considered when patients with thyrotoxicosis are treated in this way. Four main types of carcinoma are described. (1) *Papillary carcinoma* affects a younger age group than the other patterns of carcinoma. The primary tumour is often very small but it metastasizes early to cervical lymph nodes. Because the primary tumour may be undetectable clinically, these metastases have been erroneously called 'lateral aberrant thyroid'. In spite of early lymph node metastases, these tumours often remain confined to the neck and have a relatively good prognosis. (2) *Follicular carcinoma.* This resembles, sometimes very closely, normal thyroid gland. It shows a greater tendency to spread by way of the blood stream, especially to the lungs and bones. It is this pattern of tumour which is best suited to radioiodine therapy. Initial total thyroidectomy is required to stimulate TSH production by the pituitary. This causes increased functional activity by the metastases so that they take up a therapeutic dose of radioiodine. If significant quantities of thyroid tissue remain in the neck, these concentrate the administered iodine and insufficient radioiodine is taken up by metastases to produce a therapeutic effect. (3) *Anaplastic carcinoma.* This may either be of small cell or giant cell pattern. They are rapidly growing tumours which metastasize readily by lymphatics and blood stream. Most do not concentrate iodine and so are not amenable to radioiodine therapy. The prognosis is poor. Small cell carcinoma may be confused with primary malignant lymphoma of the thyroid. (4) *Medullary carcinoma.* This arises from parafollicular cells and does not produce colloid. It occurs over a wide age range and has a variable prognosis. It shows accumulation of amyloid. Some of these tumours are familial and there may be associated lesions such as muco-cutaneous polyps and adrenal phaeochromocytoma.

The Parathyroid Glands

The parathyroid glands impinge on the clinical scene as a result of either under-production or over-production of parathormone. The commonest cause of underactivity leading to tetany is ablation, usually as a complication of thyroidectomy. Overactivity can arise spontaneously, or secondarily to the usual stimulus for parathormone production, i.e. a low serum calcium. In clinical practice, the latter is most commonly due to impaired phosphate excretion as a result of chronic renal disease, and leads to hyperplasia of all the glands. Spontaneous or primary overactivity is most commonly a consequence of a functioning adenoma in one of the glands or rarely it is due to primary hyperplasia or carcinoma. An independently functioning adenoma can occasionally develop in secondary hyperplasia (tertiary hyperparathyroidism). Adenomas vary in size, averaging about 300 mg (normal total weight of four parathyroids = 120 mg) and are usually of orange brown colour. Histologically they consist predominantly of dark chief cells, although some tumours are mainly oxyphil cells. A rim of normal parathyroid is compressed around the tumour. In hyperplasia the whole gland is involved due mainly to chief cell hyperplasia, and the cytoplasm of these cells may be vacuolated or 'water-clear'. The commonest effect of primary parathyroid overactivity is to cause mobilization of calcium from the bones and increased excretion of calcium and phosphate by the kidneys. The mobilization of calcium causes hypercalcaemia and metastatic calcification in organs such as the kidneys, with the formation of renal calculi. The bones become diffusely decalcified (osteomalacia). Histologically, seams of uncalcified bone matrix, osteoid, may be found covering the bone trabeculae. Less commonly there may be focal destruction of bone due to osteoclast activity. Haemorrhage and cyst formation occur with fibrous replacement of the destroyed bone. Many osteoclasts are found in the lesions. These changes produce the 'brown tumours' of osteitis fibrosa cystica (von Recklinghausen's disease of bone) which may be misdiagnosed as giant cell tumours of bone (osteoclastoma).

The Adrenal Glands

It is convenient to consider the adrenal as consisting of two independent endocrine glands, the cortex and the medulla. The cortex is divided into three zones, an outer zona glomerulosa, an intermediate zona fasciculata and an inner zona reticularis. These zones react differently in various pathological states. Diseases of the cortex may either result in increased or decreased function.

Decreased Cortical Activity

Acute cortical insufficiency may result from massive bilateral adrenal haemorrhage causing destruction of the whole cortex. This is found as a complication of severe infection, particularly meningococcal septicaemia (Waterhouse–Friderichsen syndrome). There is often evidence of intravascular thrombosis similar to that which may be produced in the generalized Shwartzman phenomenon.

Chronic cortical insufficiency leads to the development of *Addison's disease* in which there is skin pigmentation, wasting, weakness and hypotension. There may be anorexia, nausea and vomiting. There is loss of sodium in the urine leading to hyponatraemia and uraemia. Tuberculosis was the commonest cause of chronic cortical insufficiency in the past but with the reduction in the number of cases of tuberculosis, this has become less important. Chronic cortical insufficiency is now more commonly due to primary atrophy. The latter is an autoimmune disease in which there is lymphocytic infiltration of the cortex, with destruction of cortical cells and fibrous replacement. Some cases of primary atrophy also have antibodies to thyroid and gastric parietal cells. Hypopituitarism, secondary carcinoma and amyloidosis are less common causes of Addison's disease.

Increased Cortical Activity

Increased cortical activity may result in excessive production of one or more of the three main hormone groups, the C21 steroids (cortisol, corticosterone, and aldosterone) the C19 steroids (androgens) and the C18 steroids (oestrogens). The associated structural changes may be bilateral hyperplasia, adenoma or carcinoma.

The adrenogenital syndrome when due to bilateral hyperplasia is the result of an enzyme block whereby the adrenal is unable to synthesize normal quantities of cortisol. This causes the pituitary to produce more ACTH which further stimulates the adrenal to produce more androgens. The clear cells of the zona fasciculata of the cortex become replaced by compact cells similar to those of the zona reticularis. Treatment with cortisol reduces the pituitary stimulation with reduction in output of C_{19} steroids by the adrenal. Congenital adrenogenital syndrome causes pseudohermaphroditism due to the effect of virilizing hormones on the external genitalia. In postnatal life, the adrenogenital syndrome may be due to hyperplasia or tumour, the latter functioning independently of the pituitary are therefore not suppressed by cortisol. All cases of adrenogenital syndrome show virilism.

Cushing's syndrome is characterized by obesity, mainly of the trunk, plethora, skin striae, hypertension, osteoporosis and diabetes mellitus. It may be due to predominant secretion of C21 steroids or there may be a mixture of C_{21} and C_{19} steroids in which case virilism will also be present. Most adult cases are due to bilateral cortical hyperplasia due to overstimulation by the pituitary. Some of these cases show small basophil adenomas of the pituitary and in a few there may be chromophobe pituitary adenomas. In children, and less commonly in adults, adenoma or carcinoma of the adrenal cortex may be the primary pathology. In these cases there is independent function by the tumour producing large quantities of cortisol which suppresses ACTH production by the pituitary causing atrophy of the contralateral adrenal cortex. Bilateral hyperplasia of the cortex and Cushing's syndrome may also be caused by corticotrophin produced by bronchial oat cell carcinoma.

Primary aldosteronism (Conn's syndrome) is due to an adenoma or hyperplasia of the zona glomerulosa of the adrenal cortex. The adenomata are golden yellow and rarely exceed 1 cm diameter. Aldosterone causes sodium retention and potassium wastage in the urine. There is hypertension and profound weakness due to hypokalaemia. Aldosterone is not secreted under the influence of pituitary trophic hormones, but the zona glomerulosa is stimulated to produce aldosterone by angiotensin which is formed by the action of renin on angiotensinogen in blood. Renin is found in the juxtaglomerular cells of the afferent arteriole in renal glomeruli. Abnormalities of renin production may therefore cause secondary hyperplasia of the adrenal zona glomerulosa (secondary aldosteronism).

Overproduction of oestrogen by the adrenal is rare and usually associated with cortical carcinoma. It causes precocious puberty in girls and feminization in men.

Cortical adenoma is a common finding at post-mortem and most appear to be without clinical hormonal effect. They are usually less than 1 cm diameter and golden yellow in colour. Histologically they are composed of pale cells resembling those found in the zona fasciculata.

Cortical carcinoma is usually much larger than adenoma. It may show pleomorphism and mitotic activity, but often these tumours mimic adenomas in their histological appearance. Invasion, necrosis and haemorrhage are all sinister features. They metastasize by the blood stream to the lungs and the prognosis is poor.

Reduced Medullary Activity

No syndrome can be attributed to diminished medullary function. This is not surprising for removal of both adrenals necessitates supplements of cortical steroids only.

Increased Medullary Activity

Phaeochromocytoma. Increased medullary activity is produced pathologically most frequently by a tumour of the noradrenaline and adrenaline secreting cells, the phaeochromocytoma. This is usually benign, its average size being that of a plum, though occasionally it may be much larger. Its cut surface may be cystic and haemorrhagic, and usually turns strikingly dark brown on exposure to air. The cells have an affinity for chrome salts (chromaffin). Histologically the tumour shows the presence of large cells, with abundant pink granular cytoplasm loosely arranged round a sinusoidal network. The tumour is one of the less common known causes of hypertension but is nevertheless an important one because its removal leads to cure in early cases. Rarely, phaeochromocytoma may arise in the sympathetic chain outside the adrenal.

Non-functioning Tumours. These are usually taken to include neuroblastoma and ganglioneuroma although occasionally these may be associated with hypertension. Neuroblastoma is a tumour of infancy and childhood being uncommon above the age of seven. It is frequently haemorrhagic and consists of immature neural tissue arranged in sheets or rosettes. Some neuroblastomas mature to ganglioneuromas; this is more likely with congenital tumours. Most are highly malignant and metastasize by the blood stream to bone and liver, by lymphatics to regional lymph nodes and by direct invasion of surrounding structures. Ganglioneuromas occur more frequently in the sympathetic chain but 10 per cent occur in the adrenal medulla. They are firm, fibrous tumours, usually encapsulated. Histologically they consist of bundles of fibrous tissue with foci of mature ganglion cells. These tumours are benign although transitional forms to neuroblastoma may be found.

Secondary Carcinoma

The adrenal is one of the commonest sites for metastatic carcinoma especially from primary carcinoma in the bronchus. In spite of massive replacement of the gland they rarely give symptoms of adrenal insufficiency.

Pituitary

As with the adrenal, the pituitary is best regarded as two endocrine glands, the anterior adenohypophysis which is formed from Rathke's pouch and the posterior neurohypophysis formed from the floor of the third ventricle. The adenohypophysis is made up of chromophobe cells (50 per cent) acidophil cells (40 per cent) and basophil cells (10 per cent). Mucin stains reveal that all basophils, some chromophobes and a few acidophils are mucoid cells. Various trophic hormones are produced by the adenohypophysis. Mucoid cells produce adrenocorticotrophic hormone (ACTH) thyrotrophic hormone (TSH) follicle stimulating hormone (FSH) and luteinizing hormone (LH). Acidophil cells produce growth hormone and prolactin. The neurohypophysis is the source of antidiruetic hormone (ADH) and oxytocin.

Hypopituitarism

This may result from trauma, pressure from tumours within or adjacent to the pituitary, and interference with the blood supply. In children hypopituitarism may either produce *Fröhlich's syndrome*—obesity, mental retardation and genital hypoplasia or the *Lorain-Levi syndrome*—symmetric dwarfism and genital hypoplasia. In adults, hypopituitarism is most often associated with post-partum infarction of the pituitary as a result of shock due to haemorrhage—*Sheehan's syndrome*. This may become manifest by a failure of lactation and subsequently of continued amenorrhoea. There is loss of pubic axillary hair and the skin is thin and dry. Lack of growth hormone causes atrophy of organs and lack of trophic hormones causes failure of other endocrine glands, particularly the thyroid and later the adrenal cortex.

Failure of the neurohypophysis results in *diabetes insipidus* due to lack of ADH. This causes polyuria and polydipsia.

Hyperpituitarism

Acromegaly is due to an acidophil adenoma producing excess growth hormone. There is enlargement of the jaw, hands and feet, coarsening of the skin, enlargement of other organs such as liver, kidneys and heart, and diabetes mellitus. Before fusion of epihyses, excessive secretion of growth hormone results in *gigantism.*

Cushing's syndrome may be associated with a small basophil adenoma of the pituitary; less commonly a chromophobe adenoma, composed of mucoid cells, may be the cause. These tumours cause excessive secretion of ACTH resulting in bilateral cortical hyperplasia of the adrenal.

Inappropriate secretion of antidiuretic hormone may be due to tumours outside the neurohypophysis, notably oat cell carcinoma of the bronchus.

Tumours

Tumours of the anterior pituitary are adenomas derived from chromophobe, acidophil or basophil cells. Chromophobe tumours are usually non-functional unless they consist of mucoid cells; by compression of surrounding tissue they may cause hypopituitarism. The largest adenomas are chromophobe; basophil adenomas are usually microscopic in size. *Rathke's pouch cysts* occur between the anterior and posterior parts of the pituitary causing pressure effects on these structures. The cysts are lined by ciliated epithelium.

Craniopharyngiomas are derived from remnants of Rathke's pouch. They may be cystic or solid and composed of squamous epithelium or they may resemble adamantinoma of the jaw. They are slow growing, locally malignant tumours, found most often above the pituitary.

Gliomas may arise in the neurohypophysis but are rare. *Meningio-*

mas may occur in the vicinity of the pituitary fossa and mimic pituitary tumours.

Secondary carcinoma in the pituitary is seen commonly in patients undergoing hypophysectomy for advanced breast carcinoma. There may be direct infiltration of the pituitary from nasopharyngeal carcinomas.

Further Reading

Symington, T. (1970) *Functional Pathology of the Human Adrenal Gland*. Edinburgh, Livingstone.

26 Diseases of the Haemopoietic and Allied Systems

The diseases discussed in this chapter fall mainly into four groups, the anaemias, the myeloproliferative disorders, the malignant lymphomas and haemorrhagic diseases.

The Anaemias

Anaemia is the state when the circulating red cell mass is less than normal, and is diagnosed by the finding of a lower than normal haemoglobin level in the blood. The red cells are formed in the bone marrow from their nucleated precursors, the normoblasts, and when mature, find their way into the blood stream, where they remain on an average for 120 days. The ageing cells are then taken up by the cells of the reticulo-endothelial system to be broken down as already described on p. 19.

Anaemia can therefore result from (1) a decreased output of red cells from the bone marrow (marrow failure), (2) a shorter time in the circulation ('short cell life'), or (3) a combination of (1) and (2).

(a) *Marrow Failure*

(i) This may be due to aplasia of erythropoietic tissue, e.g. in idiopathic aplastic anaemia, or following exposure to ionizing radiations, or after poisoning with some drugs, e.g. chloramphenicol.

(ii) It may be the result of the lack of an essential nutrient for red cell formation, e.g. iron (iron deficiency anaemia) vitamin B_{12} (pernicious anaemia) and folic acid (idiopathic steatorrhoea).

(iii) It may follow the crowding out of erythropoietic tissue by tumour cells, as in secondary carcinoma and the leukaemias.

(b) *Short Cell Life Anaemias*

These may arise either because the circulating red cells are broken up more quickly than normal (haemolytic anaemias) or because the blood is lost in an acute haemorrhage (haemorrhagic anaemias). The haemolytic anaemias can be further subdivided on the basis that (1) the red cells are structurally defective, or (2) red cell antibodies are circulating in the blood. The best-known examples of the first group are hereditary spherocytosis and sickle cell anaemia. Rhesus haemolytic disease of the newborn and autoimmune haemolytic anaemia are examples of the second group.

(c) *Anaemias due to a Combination of Marrow Failure and Short Cell Life*

The most obvious example of this is seen in some patients with leukaemia. Red cell production is impaired by marrow proliferation of leukaemic cells and there is, not infrequently, an associated haemolytic process.

A similar state of affairs may develop in many other conditions—such as carcinomatosis and prolonged or severe sepsis.

Pathological Features of Anaemia

The Bone Marrow

This may be studied by way of biopsy during life, such as an iliac trephine or rib biopsy, or at autopsy, when the sternum, vertebral column, and femur are usually examined. The information obtained both macroscopically and microscopically is limited; and it should also be remembered that red marrow is normally more extensive in children than adults. In aplastic anaemia the red marrow usually to be seen in the adult head of the femur at autopsy is replaced by fat, and the vertebrae and sternum appear a yellowish pink. In all other primary anaemias the red marrow is more abundant than normal. This can only be detected with the naked eye in the adult at autopsy by observing that the red marrow is to be seen farther down the shaft of the femur than normal. Histologically the balance between haemopoietic and fat cells gives an indication of red cell activity. The red cell precursors can usually be distinguished from white cell precursors in the marrow, but the finer abnormalities of the red cell precursors, which are of diagnostic value, such as the change to megaloblasts in pernicious anaemia, are best diagnosed in fresh haematologically stained films. The lesions bringing about secondary anaemias such as metastatic carcinoma and leukaemia have, of course, the characteristic pathological features of those diseases.

Iron Stores

If red cell breakdown is in excess of red cell formation there will be a build-up of iron stores in the body. This most commonly occurs in haemolytic and pernicious anaemias. If the prussian blue reaction is carried out at post mortem on slices of liver and spleen, where the cells of the reticulo-endothelial system are abundant, a strongly positive reaction will be obtained in these diseases. Inability to find iron histologically anywhere in the reticulo-endothelial tissues supports a diagnosis of iron deficiency, but this examination is rarely necessary for diagnosis.

The Tissues

Anaemia is a cause of tissue anoxia. When death takes place after a severe acute anaemia, such as following a massive haemorrhage, all organs will look very pale at autopsy. If the anaemia is more chronic, such as in iron deficiency or pernicious anaemias, degenerative changes may be observed in the tissue cells, the most common of which is fatty change, macroscopically most easily observed in the liver and myocardium (see p. 29).

The Myeloproliferative Disorders

The diseases which are included under this heading have been listed earlier (p. 114). Their common factor is that they are neoplastic disorders primarily involving the bone marrow.

The Leukaemias

These are neoplastic diseases affecting the white blood cells and are sooner or later invariably fatal. They account for about 3 per cent of all deaths from malignant disease, are increasing in frequency, and may occur at all ages. Most cases exist as one of three fairly well-defined forms, acute leukaemia, chronic myeloid leukaemia and chronic lymphatic leukaemia. The aetiology of human leukaemia is still obscure. Chromosome abnormalities of many types have been detected in acute leukaemia, and of a constant type in chronic myeloid leukaemia (p. 100). Exposure to ionizing radiations is one known way by which such alterations can be brought about.

Acute Leukaemia

This form is showing the most striking increase. It is one of the commonest malignant diseases in childhood, but another peak of increasing incidence occurs in old age. It may complicate chronic myeloid leukaemia ('myeloblastic termination'). Its onset is sudden and its progress, untreated, is rapid. The bone marrow becomes packed with primitive white cells (leucoblasts), so that macroscopically the red marrow takes on a purplish hue. The replacement of fatty marrow by red marrow may not, however, be extensive, presumably because of the short duration of disease before death. The leucoblasts also appear in the blood, though in variable numbers. Evidence of leukaemic proliferation in extra-medullary sites may be present, but is uncommonly extensive. The spleen may be slightly enlarged and some of the lymph nodes may be swollen and of purplish colour. Acute leukaemia causes rapid deterioration of the patient chiefly because of its effect on haemopoiesis. Rapidly progressive anaemia is common, and is reflected in the pallor of the viscera observed at autopsy. Purpura, consisting of small haemorrhages (petechiae and ecchymoses (bruises), is also frequently observed, as a result of the thrombocytopenia which develops. The ulceration of mucous membranes, especially within the mouth, is probably in part due to the severe reduction of neutrophil polymorphs which occurs in this disease (neutropenia, agranulocytosis).

Chronic Myeloid Leukaemia

This disease is nearly as frequent as acute leukaemia and is most common in middle age. It consists of an uncontrolled proliferation of the cells of the granular series, with the result that large numbers of cells of all degrees of maturation appear in the blood stream. There is usually a great expansion of active marrow, so that at autopsy the whole shaft of the femur will be seen to contain this purplish tissue. Extramedullary proliferation of cells is usually striking, and may occur in many situations, but tends to be particularly evident in the spleen, which is usually greatly enlarged. The cut surface is swollen, soft and without architectural detail; infarcts and perisplenitis are common. The onset of the disease is more insidious than in acute leukaemia, and the interference with normal haemopoiesis less dramatic. The survival time after diagnosis is on an average about three years.

Chronic Lymphatic Leukaemia

This is a little less common than the other two variants, and tends to occur in the older age groups. It consists of an uncontrolled proliferation of lymphoid tissue with the result that large numbers of small lymphocytes are produced at these sites, and appear in the blood. It is not surprising that swelling of lymph nodes is a common and dominant feature, but other tissues containing lymphoid follicles also frequently enlarge. The bone marrow is usually packed with lymphocytes by the time the patient is first seen, and the spleen and liver are moderately enlarged. The natural history and the effects on normal haemopoiesis are similar to those of chronic myeloid leukaemia, though a higher proportion run a relatively benign course. There is usually some degree of haemolytic anaemia in these cases.

Other Myeloproliferative Disorders

Multiple myeloma

This is a disease caused by the neoplastic proliferation of plasma cells derived from one parent cell (monoclonal). Since each plasma cell is responsible for the production of a specific immunoglobulin, it follows that all plasma cells derived from one parent cell will produce the same type of immunoglobulin. The neoplastic proliferation of these cells suppresses normal plasma cells with the result that other immunoglobulins in the serum are diminished or lost. The sharp band seen on electrophoresis of serum proteins from patients with multiple myeloma indicates a monoclonal immunoglobulin. The abnormal plasma cells synthesize excess light chains (p. 13) which are excreted in the urine as Bence Jones protein. Multiple myeloma is a disease which is usually confined to the bone marrow. There is diffuse plasma cell infiltration of the marrow; foci of soft deep-red tumour destroy the bone and commonly cause pathological fractures. Histologically the tumour cells may be mature or primitive plasma cells. The kidney may be severely damaged either because of accumulation of protein in tubules with obstruction to urine flow or there may be massive deposition of amyloid in glomeruli, blood vessels and around tubules. The serum calcium is usually raised. Anaemia is common, but myeloma cells are rarely to be found in the blood. There is evidence that plasma cell proliferation takes 10 to 15 years before it causes clinical disease but following the onset of symptoms, death usually results within two years.

Myelofibrosis is a slowly progressive disease characterized by anaemia, a raised white cell count, splenomegaly, and a failure to aspirate marrow on diagnostic puncture (the 'dry tap'). The histological picture of a fibrotic marrow is characteristic, showing abnormal haemopoiesis and increased numbers of reticulum cells, including giant-cell forms. The spleen, liver and lymph nodes also show the presence of these abnormal reticulum cells, together with foci of extramedullary haemopoiesis. Many of the features are similar to those found in chronic myeloid leukaemia and there may be difficulty in distinguishing the two conditions. The Philadelphia chromosome is only found in chronic myeloid leukaemia.

Polycythaemia vera results from an insidious proliferation of red cell precursors in the marrow, which leads to an increased red cell mass in the body. Thromboses are likely through the increased viscosity of the blood. A proportion die through the development of leukaemia. Secondary polycythaemia occurs in states of chronic anoxia such as chronic lung disease, congenital heart disease and living at high altitudes. This is not included in myeloproliferative disorders.

Thrombocythaemia is a rare disease, leading to the appearance in the blood of a greatly increased number of platelets, which may be shown to have imperfect function. Both haemorrhages and thromboses develop as complications.

Erythaemia is the red cell counterpart of acute leukaemia, and is much rarer than the latter.

The Malignant Lymphomas

A striking point of difference between the malignant lymphomas and other malignant tumours is that the former are of multicentric origin, though it is probable that metastatic foci also develop as with carcinoma and other sarcomas. The lymphomatous masses are most liable to arise where the lympho-reticular tissue is most concentrated, i.e. in the lymph nodes and spleen, but as the lymphoreticular system is widespread throughout the body, malignant lymphoma can appear in almost any situation in the body.

The swollen lymph nodes are usually pale grey-brown, homogeneous, and moist on section. If other viscera are involved the tumour will show similar appearances. Histologically the common change shown by all forms of lymphoma is the finding that the normal lymph node architecture is obliterated as a result of the proliferation of tumour cells. There is a wide range of survival time but most are ultimately fatal. Lymphomas account for about 3 per cent of all deaths from malignant disease.

Various classifications have been used. Most depend on a histological classification based on the predominant cell type or types. They may be lymphocytic or lymphoblastic; 'reticulum' cells include those that are histiocytic and primitive precursors or stem cells. Tumour cells may occur as a diffuse sheet or they may be nodular, mimicking normal follicles. As a generalization, nodular lymphomas have a better prognosis than diffuse forms, and those consisting of differentiated mature lymphocytes a better prognosis than lymphoblasts or 'reticulum' cells.

Hodgkin's Disease

This is the commonest variant accounting for about half the cases. It is most common between the ages of 20 and 40 but may occur at any age. The enlarged lymph nodes tend to remain discrete and rubbery, and the spleen cut surface often presents a blotchy pale and dark brown cut surface, traditionally likened to 'hard-bake' toffee (i.e. toffee with nuts). The histological picture varies considerably from case to case, and even from node to node. There is always an increased number of large histiocytic, reticulum cells characterized by pale vesicular oval nuclei. A proportion contain two nuclei lying side by side, the so-called mirror image nuclei of the Hodgkin giant cells, also called Sternberg-Reed cells. The proportion of lymphocytes varies from case to case. Where lymphocytes predominate and reticulum cells and Sternberg-Reed cells are scanty, the disease runs a fairly benign course, often over 15 years or more. This is therefore referred to as benign Hodgkin's disease (lymphocyte predominant Hodgkin's disease or Hodgkin's paragranuloma). If there is a mixture of lymphocytes and reticulum cells, often with eosinophil leucocytes and fibroblasts forming collagen, the disease is called Hodgkin's granuloma (mixed cellularity Hodgkin's disease). This is the commonest pattern of the disease; it has a poor prognosis with only 40 per cent surviving 5 years. If reticulum cells predominate, the disease runs a rapid course with few patients surviving 5 years (lymphocyte depleted Hodgkin's disease, Hodgkin's sarcoma). One other variant is found in which a nodular pattern is emphasized by the nodules being surrounded by dense fibrous tissue. Within the nodules, the cellular picture is of the mixed cellularity pattern but in spite of this many patients with nodular sclerosing Hodgkin's disease survive for 10 years or more.

The disease may present with a generalized lymphadenopathy but it often is found as enlargement of a single lymph node or a single group of lymph nodes. Patients with active disease may have a fever which fluctuates from day to day and there may be a blood eosinophilia.

Nodular Lymphocytic Lymphoma

This occurs most frequently in those over 40 years. It presents most frequently as cervical lymphadenopathy but spreads to involve other lymph nodes. Histologically it may be difficult to distinguish from reactive hyperplasia of lymph nodes but points of importance are that the nodules occur throughout the node, they do not contain reactive germinal centres and the sinusoids become compressed and obscured. Many cases survive for 10 years or more, but eventually progress to more active forms of lymphoma. It must be emphasized, that other nodular lymphomas may consist of lymphoblasts or reticulum cells and these do not have as favourable a prognosis.

Lymphosarcoma

This term is often used to describe both diffuse lymphocytic and diffuse lymphoblastic lymphoma. The former should be separated as the better differentiation has a much more favourable prognosis. Lymphoblastic lymphosarcoma can occur at any age, but is most common in the elderly. At clinical presentation there is usually widespread lymph node enlargement with rapid progression causing necrosis and haemorrhage. The bone marrow may be infiltrated and lymphosarcoma cells may escape into the peripheral blood. Few of these patients survive 5 years.

Reticulum Cell Sarcoma

This may be either histiocytic or stem cell, nodular or diffuse. Nodular histiocytic lymphoma has a more favourable prognosis than other forms of reticulum sell sarcoma but not as good as nodular lymphocytic tumours. Reticulum cell sarcoma occurs most commonly in the elderly and presents with generalized lymphadenopathy. An important form of presentation is tonsillar enlargement or 'tonsillitis'. For this reason tonsillitis should be treated with caution in the elderly especially if unilateral. The morc aggressive forms of reticulum cell sarcoma have a very poor prognosis with few patients surviving two years.

Organ Lymphoma

Any of the histological patterns of lymphoma already described may occur, apparently as primary disease, in organs such as thyroid, stomach, intestine, testis, etc. Disease in these cases often is confined to the organ and may be successfully treated by surgery and local radiotherapy. They eventually spread, first to regional lymph nodes and eventually as disseminated malignant lymphoma.

Thymus

The relationship of the thymus to immunity has already been indicated (p. 87). Thymic *hypoplasia* is found in children of both sexes and is apparently inherited as a recessive gene. These children show agammaglobulinaemia, failure of development of lymphoid tissue and a susceptibility to infection. Thymic *hyerplasia* is found in a variety of conditions, some of which are accepted as being autoimmune diseases. They include Graves' disease, primary atrophy of the adrenal, myasthenia gravis and disseminated lupus erythematosus. In some children, sudden death is associated with thymic hyperplasia and has been called status thymicolymphaticus. Most of these children probably die from overwhelming infection, although adrenocortical insufficiency may account for others.

Thymomas may be benign or malignant, but even the latter are only locally infiltrative and rarely metastasize. They may mimic either the lymphoid component of the thymus or the epithelial component. Mixtures of the two give an appearance very like Hodgkin's disease called granulomatous thymoma. About 40 per cent of patients with a thymoma show features of myasthenia gravis (p. 287). Some of these patients have improvement in their myasthenia following excision of the tumour. Other cases of thymoma are associated with haemopoietic abnormality, particularly red cell aplasia.

It may be impossible to distinguish between malignant lymphoma or secondary carcinoma in lymph nodes in the anterior mediastinum and thymoma. Some cases of Cushing's syndrome reported as being due to thymoma are probably due to metastatic oat cell carcinoma of lung which has a well-recognized association with this syndrome.

Teratoma may occur in the anterior mediastinum but there is doubt as to whether it actually arises in the thymus. These tumours may be benign or malignant. In some there may be a seminoma pattern similar to that found in the testis.

Haemorrhagic Disorders

Bleeding and coagulation disorders are not infrequent. The former are gathered together under the name *purpura* by which is meant the existence of a clinical syndrome in which there are small (petechial) haemorrhages in skin, mucous membranes and endothelial surfaces (pp. 36, 37). The purpuras fall into two main classes, according to whether platelet deficiency, or thrombocytopenia, is present or not. Important causes of thrombocytopenia are leukaemia, aplastic anaemia, malignant lymphoma, disseminated lupus erythematosis, severe infection, irradiation and cytotoxic drugs. Allergic vasculitis, including Henoch-Schönlein purpura is an important non-thrombocytopenic cause. Thrombocytopenic purpuras are usually the more severe forms. *Haemophilia* is the best-known disease due to defect of blood coagulation, and results from an hereditary absence of antihaemophilic globulin, occurring in males (p. 98). Haemorrhage in these cases most frequently occurs into joints or soft tissues; it may complicate surgery or trauma by a continuous slow ooze from the wound. Correction of the deficiency requires fresh (or fresh-frozen) plasma, cryoprecipitate, or whole blood. A purified preparation of antihaemophilic globulin can be prepared from animal sources, but it may be used only in an emergency, as antibodies readily develop after its administration. Other coagulation disorders include congenital deficiency of Factor IX (Christmas disease) and acquired deficiencies of Factors V and VII in liver disease. Circulating anti-coagulants may produce a similar clinical effect.

Further Reading

Gruchy, G. C. de (1970) *Clinical Haematology in Medical Practice.* 3rd edn. Oxford, Blackwell.

Rappaport, H. (1966) *Atlas of Tumour Pathology* Section III, Fascicle 8, Tumours of the Haemopoietic System. Washington D.C., AFIP.

27 | The Skeletal System

The Joints

Acute Arthritis

This may be bacterial in origin, developing through an open wound or by way of the blood stream. In some cases suppuration may take place. The organisms most likely to cause the disease are the pyogenic cocci. Acute inflammation may also occur as a feature of some of the collagen diseases, such as rheumatic fever and anaphylactoid purpura, but in these instances mononuclear cells, rather than polymorphs, predominate.

Chronic Bacterial Arthritis

This may develop as a sequel of acute arthritis, or may be due to tuberculosis or syphilis. It is now a much rarer disease than it was at the beginning of the century, and this improvement is in large measure due to the success of antibiotic therapy.

Osteoarthritis

This is a common disease starting usually in late adult life, is insidious in onset, and chronic in progress. Men are more often affected than women, and the larger joints, especially the hip-joint, are most frequently involved, giving rise to pain and limitation of movement. The aetiology is obscure; trauma may be an important initiating factor but the disease is commonly considered to be a degenerative process, first of cartilage and then bone. The joint cartilage loses its basophilia because mucopolysaccharides leak out. This reveals fibrillation of the matrix, the fibrils running at right angles to the articular surface. The surface cartilage splits along the fibrils and becomes roughened. Gradually it is worn away, exposing the underlying compact bone, which becomes smooth and hard due to new bone formation, and in places the surface is grooved. Beneath the sclerotic bone, trabeculae become osteoporotic and there is an excess of soft fibrous marrow with cysts in between, so that the bone may collapse at one or two points. New bone formation also takes place at the margin of the articular cartilage leading to projections or osteophytes which are usually capped by fibro-cartilage. Villous projections may develop from the synovial membrane, consisting mainly of somewhat vascular fatty tissue, in which inflammatory cells are insignificant. Ankylosis or fusion of the joint surfaces does not take place.

Small bony projections on the terminal phalanges of the digits are common in old people (Heberden's nodes). They are disfiguring and may interfere with joint movement. Many regard them as mild foci of osteoarthritis, but this is by no means certain.

Rheumatoid Arthritis

The essential features of the joint changes have been described previously (p. 94). A similar arthritis is found in some patients with psoriasis and Reiter's syndrome (p. 234).

Ankylosing Spondylitis

The ligaments of the vertebrae in this disease undergo progressive ossification so that the movements of the spine become much reduced and eventually absent. The changes may involve the posterior intervertebral, costovertebral, and sacro-iliac joints. The patients have a characteristic bowed and rigid posture. The disease appears to be allied to rheumatoid arthritis.

Spinal Osteophytosis

This disease is often misdiagnosed as spinal osteoarthritis. The osteophytes develop around vertebral bodies due to expansion of intervertebral discs as a result of degenerative disc disease. Osteoarthritis, being a disease of synovial joints, never affects the vertebral bodies. It may, however, affect the posterior intervertebral joints.

Tumours

Synoviomas may be benign or malignant; they may arise from the joints or from tendon sheaths. *Benign synoviomas* occur particularly on the fingers and present as firm, brown nodules. About 20 per cent of these tumours recur after excision. A similar histological appearance is found in *pigmented villo-nodular synovitis* which is believed to be a reactive proliferation of synovial tissue affecting principally the knee joint. *Malignant synoviomas* (synoviosarcomas) are rare tumours which occur usually in the larger joints of the lower limbs. They are destructive tumours and metastasize readily to the lungs.

The Bones

Bones have three main functions: (a) the formation of a rigid framework for the body, (b) the participation in the calcium and phosphorus metabolism of the body, and (c) the housing of the haemopoietic tissue. The disturbance of some of these functions has been considered in earlier chapters. The remainder will be mentioned here.

Metabolic Bone Disease

Bone consists of a fibrous matrix, osteoid, impregnated with a form of calcium phosphate. It is a labile tissue even in adults, calcium and phosphorus being laid down or absorbed according to need. Osteoblasts are cuboidal cells lying close to the bone surface and are concerned mainly with bone formation. Osteoclasts are multinucleated giant cells scattered here and there close to the bone surface. They are active in absorption of bone and there are often notches in the bone adjacent to where they lie. Serum alkaline phosphatase activity is increased usually when there is increase of osteoblastic activity but the correlation is not exact. When studying bones histologically for evidence of metabolic activity, it has to be remembered that the usual preparations have been decalcified in order that they may be soft enough to cut. In other words they consist of osteoid. If it is required to determine how much calcium phosphate complex is present in the osteoid, undecalcified sections have to be prepared, a difficult technical procedure. Metabolic bone disease falls into two main groups: (1) disturbances in the osteoblast–osteoclast balance, and (2) disturbances in the osteoid-calcium phosphate relationship. The important examples of group (1) are osteoporosis, osteosclerosis, osteitis fibrosa cystica (hyperparathyroidism) and osteitis deformans (Paget's disease). Group (2) consists in the main of the various manifestations of osteomalacia and rickets.

Osteoporosis

This consists of a reduction in the amount of bone without change in its chemical composition, i.e. the bone is of normal texture, but there is less of it. Osteoporosis may be generalized or localized. The generalized form may be primary or secondary to endocrine disorders such as hyperthyroidism, the post-menopausal state and Cushing's syndrome. It may also be due to deficiency of protein or vitamin C (scurvy), the latter vitamin being necessary for the synthesis of the collagen matrix of bone. Examples of causes of localized osteoporosis are immobilization of the affected bone, malignant tumours, and rheumatoid arthritis. For long it has been assumed that reduced bone formation was the important factor in the development of osteoporosis, but recent evidence has indicated that a long drawn-out, slightly increased bone resorption may be as important. A precise pathological diagnosis of the disease is difficult, because it is dependent on proving that the total mass of bone examined, though of normal texture, is of less volume than the normal counterpart. If the trabeculae of cancellous bone appear scanty and very thin, then the diagnosis is likely to be correct. The blood chemistry is normal.

Osteosclerosis

This is an increase in the amount of bone of normal chemical composition. The best-known causes are osteosclerotic secondary carcinoma such as from prostate and breast, and hypertrophic osteoarthopathy which is a complication of cardiac and respiratory disorders. Because of the increased osteoblastic activity the serum alkaline phosphatase may be increased in some cases.

Osteitis Fibrosa Cystica

This develops in hyperparathyroidism (p. 260) and displays increased osteoclast activity (bone resorption). The bone resorption is accompanied by the deposition of fibrous tissue and there is haemorrhage and cyst formation in these foci of weakened bone. Pathological fractures may occur. This fully-developed picture is rare but widespread loss of calcium from the skeleton is common in hyperparathyroidism.

Paget's Disease of Bone (*Osteitis Deformans*)

This fairly common disease of old people is of unknown aetiology. It may be widespread through the skeleton or localized to one bone. The bone is thickened, spongy and vascular. It is softer than normal and bends with weight-bearing. Thickening of the bones results in compression of nerves passing through foramina in the skull and vertebral column causing pain and loss of function. The increased vascularity of the bones may have an effect similar to an arterio-venous aneurysm, causing a high cardiac output with subsequent cardiac failure. Histologically the bones show increased osteoclastic resorption of normal dense cortical bone and osteoblastic deposition of abnormal trabeculae of new bone. This is deposited in an irregular fashion as shown by the mosaic pattern of cement lines. The medullary cavity is replaced by vascular fibrous tissue. Osteosarcoma develops in up to 10 per cent of cases and represents 30 per cent of all malignant primary tumours of bone over the age of 50.

Osteomalacia and Rickets

The same pathological process operates in these two diseases, the differences that arise being attributable to the fact that rickets develops in the actively growing bones of childhood, whereas osteomalacia is the adult counterpart. The essential defect is that the osteoid stroma of the bone becomes imperfectly impregnated with calcium and phosphate, because there is an insufficient supply of these salts to the bones. The commonest cause of this in the old days was lack of vitamin D in the diet, but this is very rare now, and as a result the diseases are much less common. Interference of absorption of vitamin D, calcium and phosphorus as a result of intestinal diseases, especially steatorrhoea, now accounts for a number of cases; most of the remainder result from renal diseases which lead to secondary hyperparathyroidism. Lack of calcium salts results in the bones being softer than normal. This is seen particularly in weight-bearing bones where deformity may be great. In children, the epiphyseal lines become widened and irregular as the cartilage cells survive for longer than normal. There is failure of provisional calcification in this cartilage. Capillaries grow into the cartilage from the metaphyseal end of the bone and bring with them osteoblasts which form osteoid. This also fails to calcify. Rickets is therefore best diagnosed by observing the wide, poorly ossifying, epiphyseal lines seen on X-ray; it can also be studied by costo-chrondral biopsy. The histological diagnosis of osteomalacia is dependent on demonstrating 'osteoid seams' at the edge of bone trabeculae in undecalcified sections.

Inflammation of Bones

Osteomyelitis

This disease is much less common than before the days of antibiotic therapy, when it used to cause a high mortality and morbidity. The disease consists of a blood-borne infection generally with *Staphylococcus aureus*, starting towards the end of the shaft of a long bone (metaphysis) usually in young people. Suppuration results and, without active surgical drainage, is liable to spread both down the shaft of the bone and outwards, separating the periosteum from the underlying cortex. As a result, much of the bone becomes necrotic forming a 'sequestrum', which acts as a foreign body unless it is removed surgically or discharged spontaneously. The spontaneous discharge is often rendered difficult because the stripped periosteum starts to lay down new bone often called an 'involucrum', which encases the sequestrum albeit incompletely. Septicaemia may cause death within a few days. The long drawn-out suppuration following sequestrum formation used to be a frequent cause of amyloid disease. Extension into joints is uncommon.

Tuberculosis of Bones and Joints

This is again a disappearing disease because of improved nutrition and specific antibiotic therapy. It was in previous years an important cause of ill-health among the young. It is predominantly blood-borne, and in the old days, an appreciable fraction of cases were due to bovine tubercle bacilli ingested in infected milk. The joints may be involved primarily, or secondarily from bone, the avascular cartilage being no bar to the spread of tuberculosis in contrast to the situation in acute osteomyelitis. Tubercles develop which lead to resorption and necrosis of bone and cartilage and disorganization of the joint cavity. Collapse and fracture of infected bone may occur, and the accumulating caseous material may spread into the surrounding tissues. The kyphosis and scoliosis of the spine resulting from tuberculous infection is often termed 'Pott's disease', and this may cause compression of the spinal cord and paraplegia. The local spread of infection from the vertebrae may track along the psoas muscle and present as a 'cold abscess' below the inguinal ligament.

Syphilis of Bones and Joints

This is again chiefly of historical interest. Osteochondritis can form part of congenital syphilis. Chronic periostitis and gummatous necrosis are the commoner manifestations of tertiary syphilis, the former resulting in new bone formation giving, among other changes, 'sabre tibia' and the latter leading to the formation of cavities within the bone, the cranium and hard palate being relatively frequently involved.

Histiocytosis X

Eosinophilic granuloma is of unknown aetiology but it has the appearances of an inflammatory reaction. It causes destruction and expansion of bone particularly in children. Local excision is usually curative. There are features of similarity with Hand-Schüller-Christian disease (p. 35) and Letterer-Siwe disease, so that the three are often grouped together under the term Histiocytosis X.

Fractures

The processes involved in the repair of fractured bones have already been briefly outlined (p. 23).

Tumours

Secondary tumours, usually carcinomas, are much commoner than primary malignant tumours of bone. Certain carcinomas show a predilection for metastasizing to bone and these include carcinoma of the lung, breast, prostate, thyroid and kidney.

Primary Tumours of Bone: Benign

Osteoid Osteoma is a tumour of adolescents and young adults. It occurs in the shaft of long bones and presents as bone pain. Radiologically the lesion is osteolytic surrounded by a rim of sclerotic bone. It consists of immature, woven bone and osteoid matrix. A similar, but larger lesion may be found in vertebrae and is called *benign osteoblastoma*. *Exostosis* develops from *ecchondroma* by ossification. These are developmental abnormalities rather than true tumours. They arise on the outer aspect of long bones near the epiphyseal cartilage and may produce large masses that limit movement of adjacent joints. They rarely become malignant. Multiple ecchondromata and exostoses are called diaphyseal aclasis which is inherited as a dominant gene.

Enchondroma is a cartilage tumour occurring most commonly in the shaft of long bones, the metacarpals, metatarsals and phalanges often being involved. Tumours occurring in the distal part of the limb almost never become malignant but tumours in the humerus, femur or limb girdles may do so, forming chondrosarcoma.

Fibrous dysplasia of bone may present as a tumour but is another developmental abnormality. It consists of fibrous tissue arranged in a whorled pattern and contains spicules of woven bone. The lesion may be single or multiple, the latter sometimes associated with skin pigmentation and precocious puberty, especially in females, giving *Albright's syndrome*.

Other benign tumours in bone include angiomas and neurofibromas similar to their counterpart in soft tissues.

Giant cell tumour of bone (*osteoclastoma*) falls between benign and malignant tumours. After local excision, about half of these tumours behave as benign neoplasms but of the remainder two-thirds will be locally invasive and one-third metastasize to lungs. Osteoclastomas rarely occur under the age of 20. They are found in the ends of long bones as osteolytic lesions which may show pathological fracture. The tumour has two components, a multinucleate giant cell resembling osteoclasts and a background spindle cell. It is this background cell which is the best guide to malignancy as assessed by mitotic activity and pleomorphism.

Primary Tumours of Bone: Malignant

Although primary malignant tumours of bone account for only 1 per cent of deaths from malignancy they are relatively common amongst sarcomas especially in children. By far the most important and the commonest is *osteosarcoma*. This occurs most frequently in the second decade of life, although Paget's disease of bone gives rise to some cases in later life. The tumours occur most frequently around the growing ends of long bones, particularly those around the knee. They may be osteolytic or osteosclerotic. The periosteum is raised by the expanding tumour, and this periosteum lays down new bone. Histologically there may be a mixture of cartilage, fibrous tissue and bone but in all osteosarcomas there is evidence of osteoid formation by malignant cells. Osteosarcomas metastasize readily by the blood stream to the lungs and there is a very poor 5-year survival. A variant, known as *parosteal osteosarcoma*, grows from the external surface of the bone and is usually very well differentiated. It is separated from the others because of its better prognosis.

Chondrosarcoma occurs later in life than osteosarcoma and affects the proximal ends of long bones, the limb girdles and ribs. The tumour consists entirely of cartilage and this shows all degrees of differentiation. These tumours are more slow growing than osteosarcoma and usually can be treated locally, although eventually some may metastasize to lungs.

Ewing's tumour is a tumour of childhood and arises from the medullary cavity of the bone. It is non-osteogenic and consists of small, dark-staining cells which destroy the bone. When the bone expands there may be some reactive (not tumorous) periosteal new bone formation. The tumour is rapidly growing and metastasizes by the blood stream to lungs, liver and to other parts of the skeleton. It may be difficult to distinguish these tumours from metastatic neuroblastoma.

Reticulum cell sarcoma may arise as a primary tumour of the medullary cavity in adults. It is probably related to Ewing's tumour in children. There is destruction of bone but these tumours are not as aggressive as osteosarcomas nor as Ewing's tumour and they may show a good response to radiotherapy. Other forms of malignant lymphoma and leukaemia may affect the bones, but usually in these there is evidence of widespread disease. Myeloma has already been discussed (p. 271).

Malignant tumours of bone also include fibrosarcoma arising from periosteum or nerve sheath, liposarcoma and angiosarcoma.

Chordoma is a locally malignant tumour that arises from the remains of the notochord. It occurs in older individuals at the lower or upper end of the vertebral column and consists of gelatinous masses of tissue with areas of haemorrhage and necrosis. Metastases are rare.

Adamantinoma is a tumour found mainly in the lower jaw and is formed from the enamel organ of teeth. It consists of islands of epithelial cells in a fibrous stroma, the outer layers of the islands being columnar or cuboidal, resembling basal cell carcinoma and the inner layers being loose textured pale cells—the stellate reticulum. These tumours are locally infiltrative and destructive, causing expansion of bone but they rarely metastasize.

Voluntary Muscles

Atrophy

Atrophy of muscles takes place if they are immobilized, if there has been prolonged bed rest, or if there is paralysis of the nerve of supply. It may also follow inanition or cachexia, and is a prominent feature of primary muscle diseases (myopathies).

Hypertrophy

This can follow exercise; it may be compensatory following atrophy of adjacent muscle fibres in neuromuscular diseases.

Myositis Ossificans

This state is liable to develop if there has been haematoma formation in traumatized muscle near to bone, and consists of ectopic ossification in the organizing lesion.

Myopathies

These are a group of congenital disorders, often genetically controlled, affecting different groups of muscles, and leading to progressive weakness and ultimately death. Histologically a number of degenerative changes occur in individual muscle fibres and there may be accompanying inflammation. The distinction between myopathies and myositis may therefore be difficult. Myopathies can usually be distinguished from neural atrophy in which damaged nerves and whole bundles of atrophic muscle fibres can be seen. An increase of fat may be present among the atrophied muscle fibres.

Myasthenia Gravis

Myasthenia gravis leads to marked muscular weakness as a result of an abnormal response of the motor end-plates in the muscle to acetylcholine. There may be abnormal production or destruction of acetylcholine. The muscle weakness can be abolished by the administration of prostigmine. Collections of lymphocytes, lymphorrhages, are found in the muscle. In half the cases there is hyperplasia of the thymus and in 10 per cent of cases there is a thymoma.

Myositis

Inflammation of muscle may be associated with a neighbouring pyogenic infection or it may be due to tuberculosis, sarcoid, virus infections, parasites, or 'collagen diseases' such as dermatomyositis, scleroderma, polyarteritis nodosa or rheumatoid arthritis.

Tumours

These are rare. *Rhabdomyoma* may be found in cardiac muscle but primary neoplasms of voluntary muscle are all malignant. Rhabdomyosarcomas are of two types, embryonal and adult. Embryonal rhabdomyosarcoma occurs in young children in sites such as bladder, prostate, vagina, palate and orbit. It consists of primitive mesenchyme in which striated muscle fibres may be found. In adults, rhabdomyosarcoma may develop in large muscle masses. It produces tumours with gross nuclear pleomorphism and bizarre tumour giant cells. Both forms of rhabdomyosarcoma are highly malignant.

Further Reading

Lichtenstein, L. (1965) *Bone Tumours*. St Louis, Mosby.

28 The Central Nervous System

General Pathology

A neurone consists of nucleus and cytoplasm like other cells. The cytoplasm of the cell body contains basophilic granules of RNA (Nissl granules or tigroid substance). Cell processes, dendrites, arise from the cell body and there is a prolonged process, the axon which, with other axons, make up nerves. If the continuity of a nerve is interrupted the distal part undergoes degeneration, i.e. it swells and then becomes absorbed. Myelin sheaths break up into a number of fatty globules. The cell body also undergoes degenerative changes referred to as axonal reaction. The Nissl granules in the perinuclear cytoplasm disappear (chromatolysis), there is swelling of the cell cytoplasm and displacement of the nucleus to the periphery of the cell. If the cell dies, the nucleus undergoes karyolysis. Damaged nerve cells are capable of recovery but new ones cannot be formed. If the fibrous sheath of the distal part of the axon remains close to the proximal end, regeneration of the nerve can take place by growth of the axon from the proximal end into the distal sheath. At times, overgrowth of divided nerves and their fibrous sheaths gives rise to small, painful nodules called traumatic neuromas. Regeneration rarely happens in the brain and spinal cord where there is no neurilemmal sheath for the axon. The power of regeneration is therefore practically confined to peripheral axons.

Neuroglia forms the supporting framework of the neurones in the brain and spinal cord. It is made up of three types of cells, astrocytes, oligodendrocytes and microglia. Ependyma may also be included. Astrocytes are of two types, protoplasmic astrocytes with short branching processes found in the grey matter and fibrous astrocytes with longer processes and fewer branches found in the white matter. The long processes of fibrous astrocytes contain glial fibres. Protoplasmic astrocytes can convert to the fibrous type around sites of injury and produce these intracellular fibres (gliosis) which corresponds to fibrosis in other parts of the body. If there is extensive damage as, for example, around abscesses or haemorrhage, new vessels grow into the area and bring with them fibroblasts which lay down collagen so fibrosis may accompany gliosis. Oligodendrocytes occur around neurones and along their axons. They appear to have a nutritive function. Around damaged neurones they may swell and become more numerous—satellitosis. Microglia differs from the other glial cells in that it is not of neuroectodermal origin but is a mesodermal histiocyte. It is phagocytic and may take up lipid, becoming foamy, and referred to as a compound granular corpuscle.

Necrosis of central nervous tissue, if at all extensive and sudden, is followed by liquefaction, so that softening and ultimately cyst formation occur. Inflammatory cells of repair are derived from the blood stream. The dead tissue is phagocytosed by wandering histiocytes and microglia. Surrounding this there is a scar consisting of glial fibres and collagen.

Central nervous tissue can become oedematous. The white matter appears swollen and moist, there is widening of the gyri and flattening of the brain surface where it is compressed against the skull. Histologically the tissue appears more reticulated than normal. Rise of intracranial pressure will give papilloedema and retinal haemorrhages. There will be herniation of the cerebellar tonsils into the foramen magnum, compressing the medullary centres of respiration and circulation, herniation of the uncinate gyrus through the incisura of the tentorium cerebelli and, if there is unilateral swelling of a cerebral hemisphere, herniation of the cingulate gyrus under the falx cerebri. Herniation of the brain is more likely to occur if there is sudden rise of intracranial pressure or if cerebrospinal fluid is withdrawn by lumbar puncture.

Congenital Malformations

Anencephaly is a failure of development of the brain and is often accompanied by failure of closure of the neural tube—rachischisis—which may be partial or complete. The mildest degree of failure of closure affects only the vertebral arches usually in the lumbar region and gives rise to spina bifida occulta. The underlying cord is usually in the correct position. A meningocele occurs when failure of spinal fusion is accompanied by protrusion of the meninges, meningomyelocele when there is protrusion of the cord and meninges and syringomyelocele when there is dilatation of the spinal canal in association with the defect in the vertebral arches. Encephalocele occurs when there is a defect in the midline of the occiput. The Arnold-Chiari malformation consists of herniation of the ventero-medial portion of the cerebellum, the fourth ventricle and the medulla into the foramen magnum resulting in hydrocephalus. This malformation is often accompanied by other congenital defects such as stenosis of the aqueduct, platybasia (flattening of the base of the skull resulting in narrowing of the foramen magnum) Klippel-Feil abnormality (fusion of the cervical vertebrae) fusion of the atlas to the occiput and spina bifida. The Arnold-Chiari malformation may not become apparent until adult life.

Hydrocephalus

Cerebrospinal fluid is secreted into the lateral ventricles by the choroid plexus and circulates through the third ventricle into the fourth ventricle, from which it escapes by way of the foramina of Luschka and Magendie into the subarachnoid space. The fluid is absorbed chiefly through arachnoid granulations into the venus sinuses. Obstruction to the normal flow of cerebrospinal fluid leads to dilatation of the ventricular system—hydrocephalus. It is communicating if there is access from the ventricles to the spinal subarachnoid space but not to the cerebral subarachnoid space, i.e. the obstruction must be at the base of the brain, and non-communicating if the whole subarachnoid space is blocked from the ventricles, i.e. the obstruction must be within the ventricular system. The commonest sites of obstruction to cerebrospinal fluid circulation are the aqueduct of Sylvius and the subarachnoid space around the base of the brain. Hydrocephalus can be congenital or acquired. In the congenital form obstruction can occur at many sites, though 50 per cent arise as a result of stenosis of the aqueduct. Other causes include the Arnold-Chiari malformation and intrauterine infections such as toxoplasmosis. Tumours pressing on the aqueduct rarely give congenital hydrocephalus. The ventricles may become enormously dilated and the fontanelles of the skull widely separated. Functional disturbance may be much less than would be expected from the degree and duration of the ventricular dilatation. Acquired hydrocephalus may result from (a) pressure on the aqueduct by tumour or (b) meningitic occlusion of the arachnoid cisterns at the base of the brain. As the suture lines are often closed in this type of hydrocephalus, the brain becomes compressed against the skull and there is rapid destruction of brain tissue.

The Effects of Trauma

A number of lesions may develop from trauma. Unconsciousness can occur without evidence of any gross structural damage (concussion). With more severe injuries, damage to the brain in the form of punctate haemorrhages and oedema may be observed in two sites: (1) immediately beneath the point of impact and (2) at the diametrically opposite pole (*contre-coup*). The latter is more frequent and more severe than the former. Laceration of the brain with rupture of membranes may also occur and there may be fractures of the adjacent bone. An important form of haemorrhage is an *extradural haemorrhage* associated with rupture of a branch of the middle meningeal artery. There may be transient loss of consciousness followed by a lucid interval and then a second deepening phase of unconsciousness associated with a rise of intracranial pressure which can be relieved by timely surgical intervention.

Subdural haemorrhage may be acute or chronic. Acute haemorrhages are usually due to rupture of cortical veins often associated with laceration of the brain. Chronic subdural haematomas are due to rupture of bridging veins in the subdural space resulting in the slow leakage of blood. This undergoes organization to form a mass which compresses the brain. Chronic subdural haematomas used to be thought to be a manifestation of syphilis due to their frequency in patients with general paralysis of the insane (GPI), but these haematomas are now recognized as being traumatic. *Subarachnoid haemorrhage* may also result from trauma. *Infection* may be introduced into the cerebrospinal fluid or brain by penetrating wounds.

Intracerebral Haemorrhage

Massive cerebral haemorrhage which is a cause of 'stroke' is a common, usually progressive, and therefore fatal illness among older patients. Hypertension and atherosclerosis are the common associated conditions. The haemorrhage is found most frequently in the lentiform nucleus due to rupture of the lenticulostriate branch of the middle cerebral artery. Pontine haemorrhages may occur spontaneously or they may be secondary to cerebral haemorrhage with displacement of the brain downwards. It can be shown by microangiography that small aneurysms develop on intracerebral arteries in hypertensive patients and rupture of these arteries is believed to be the basis of cerebral haemorrhage in hypertension. Other causes of cerebral haemorrhage include trauma, angiomatous malformation, tumour, haemorrhagic diathesis, fat embolism, asphyxia, severe infections and vitamin B deficiency. The haemorrhages in many of these latter conditions are multiple and petechial.

Subarachnoid Haemorrhage

Apart from trauma, causes of subarachnoid haemorrhage are rupture of a congenital 'berry' aneurysm (p. 154) and extension of an intracerebral haemorrhage into the subarachnoid space. Rarely, mycotic or atheromatous aneurysms of the circle of Willis may rupture. Blood mixes with the cerebrospinal fluid, initially causing meningeal irritation but later causing a rise in intracranial pressure leading to coma and death. On lumbar puncture, blood-stained cerebrospinal fluid from a subarachnoid haemorrhage may be distinguished from a bloody tap due to perforation of a vertebral vein by the uniform distribution of blood and the yellow (xanthochromic) staining of the supernatent fluid after centrifugation in the former.

Cerebral Infarction

This is another common cause of 'stroke'. It is usually due to atheroma and follows occlusion of a branch of one of the cerebral arteries, often the middle cerebral artery. It may also be due to occlusion of the internal carotid artery by atheroma or thrombus. Embolism from an atheromatous plaque or from the heart, due to atrial fibrillation or mural thrombus following myocardial infarction, will have a similar result. Less commonly, cerebral infarction may be due to polyarteritis nodosa. A cerebral infarct softens quickly and eventually becomes cystic. There is gliosis around the infarcted area and slight brown staining due to haemosiderin deposition. Microscopically, degenerate tissue is seen to be phagocytosed by microglia which accumulate cytoplasmic lipid to form compound granular corpuscles. Cerebral infarction may cause death before these changes have had sufficient time to develop.

Thrombosis of spinal arteries may follow compression due to fractured vertebrae, tumour or abscess or it may be due to syphilitic endarteritis. Infarction of the spinal cord causes paraplegia due to interruption of the long tracts.

Infection of Brain and Spinal Cord

Infections of the brain, spinal cord and meninges may be due to bacteria, viruses, spirochaetes, fungi, protozoa and worms. The complications of bacterial infection are much less common than in former days because of a favourable response to early antibiotic treatment.

Suppurative Meningitis

The commonest organisms are pneumococci, meningococci and *Haemophilus influenzae*. Infection reaches the meninges through the blood stream most commonly from the lungs although infection may also spread direct from the middle ear or penetrating wounds. In pneumococcal infection, the inflammatory reaction and exudate are most noticeable over the convex surface of the cerebral hemispheres, but in other infections the base of the brain is more severely affected. Microscopically polymorphs and fibrinous exudate fill the subarachnoid space and extend around the vessels into the brain in the Virchow-Robin spaces.

Tuberculous Meningitis

Tuberculous meningitis is usually a result of miliary tuberculosis. The exudate is serofibrinous and predominantly basal. Small miliary tubercles can be identified especially along the middle cerebral artery. A small cortical 'tuberculoma'—Rich's focus—may be identified. Histologically, the tuberculous granulomata rarely contain Langhans giant cells or show caseation. There is endarteritis obliterans. Healing may leave fibrous obliteration of the subarachnoid space and result in hydrocephalus (p. 291).

Cerebral Abscess

This may result from direct spread of infection from the middle ear or paranasal air sinuses, from penetrating wounds or from blood-borne infection, especially from bronchiectasis and bacterial endocarditis. Patients present most frequently with signs of raised intracranial pressure and localizing signs according to the site involved. Macroscopically there is destruction of brain tissue with accumulation of pus and surrounding gliosis. There is progressive spread of the infection unless it is treated.

Virus Infections

Many viruses may affect the central nervous system either directly or indirectly by immunological damage. In most instances, a viraemia precedes neurological symptoms. Infection may involve predominantly the meninges (lymphocytic choriomeningitis) or the brain and spinal cord (poliomyelitis).

Lymphocytic choriomeningitis is a virus infection contracted from domestic mice. There is intense congestion of the meninges with lymphocytic infiltration. Recovery occurs in all but a few cases.

Poliomyelitis. This disease is now very much less common than in former days due largely to the success of mass vaccination. The disease may affect children or adults. Although there may be an encephalitis, it more frequently involves the spinal cord—myelitis. After an incubation period usually of 10 days, there are systemic symptoms of malaise, sore throat and vomiting and neurological manifestations of headache, stiff neck and limb pains. This is followed by flaccid paralysis of affected muscles. The infection may abort at any stage. Macroscopically the brain and cord are congested and there may be petechial haemorrhages. Microscopically the anterior horn neurones undergo degeneration and there is perivascular cuffing of the spinal vessels by polymorphs and lymphocytes. The meninges show lymphocytic infiltration. A glial scar may form in the affected area of the cord in those who survive for a prolonged period.

Viral encephalitis. A large number of viruses may cause encephalitis but they produce similar histological changes. Damage is usually most marked in the grey matter where there is degeneration of neurones and lymphocytic cuffing of vessels. Microglial cells accumulate in the inflamed area. Encephalitis due to Herpes simplex or mumps is seen infrequently in this country. Encephalitis lethargica is probably a viral infection although the virus has not been isolated. The disease occurs in epidemics and carries a high mortality. Some cases develop manifestations of parkinsonism years later. In measles and other exanthemata, perivascular demyelination may occur after one or two weeks of the infection. This appears to be an autoimmune disease similar to post-infective encephalomyelitis which can be produced experimentally in animals. It is believed that antibodies to brain tissue form and this causes demyelination. Another result of measles, which may become apparent years after infection is subacute sclerosing panencephalitis. In this condition the brain contains very large numbers of measles particles. Although there are humoral antibodies to measles in the serum, CSF and brain, there appears to be a state of impaired cell-mediated immunity (tolerance) to the measles virus.

Rabies is a virus infection transmitted by the bite of an infected animal. Quarantine of animals brought into this country has eliminated infection, but strict precautions are always required to prevent the reintroduction of the disease. The virus appears to travel along nerves to the brain and spinal cord. Aggregates of virus (Negri bodies) are found near the nucleus of infected nerve cells and are most easily seen in the hippocampus. The established disease is invariably fatal.

Herpes zoster produces a vesicular eruption in the skin in the distribution of an involved nerve. The dorsal root ganglia, or the gasserian ganglion show degeneration with accompanying inflammation. Rarely, infection may spread to the whole cord and brain stem. Herpes zoster occurs with increased frequency in patients with malignant disease especially malignant lymphomas.

Neurosyphilis

Syphilitic infection of the nervous system takes the form of (1) meningovascular syphilis and (2) parenchymatous neurosyphilis.

Meningovascular syphilis. Syphilitic meningitis usually develops within three years of the primary infection. There is chronic inflammation of the meninges over the convex surface of the cerebral hemispheres, the meninges appearing opaque. Histologically, in addition to the meningeal inflammation there is also endarteritis obliterans of the vessels. This may give small infarcts, but in the spinal cord it may lead to transverse myelitis and paraplegia.

Parenchymatous neurosyphilis occurs in two main types although these may overlap (1) tabes dorsalis and (2) general paralysis of the insane (GPI). *Tabes dorsalis* causes lightning pains in the limbs and trunk together with ataxia, loss of sensation, optic atrophy, Argyll Robertson pupils and gross osteoarthritis (Charcot's joints). There is atrophy of the dorsal columns of the spinal cord and thickening of the overlying meninges. *General paralysis* used to be one of the common diseases seen in mental institutions. The cerebral cortex becomes atrophic by a continuation of the inflammatory and vascular reaction affecting the meninges. A characteristic granular ependymitis is often present in the floor of the fourth ventricle. The clinical effects range from loss of intellect to madness. There is inco-ordination of movements and focal neurological disturbances due to cerebral infarction or trauma.

Fungal Infection

Fungal infections of the brain and meninges are rare and usually fatal. They are seen particularly in patients on immuno-suppressive therapy or with advanced malignant disease. One of the most important in this country is infection with *Cryptococcus neoformans* which produces meningitis. The meninges may be thickened and opaque, resembling tuberculous meningitis. The encapsulated organisms are usually profuse but there is little cellular reaction to them. Other fungal infections include histoplasmosis, coccidiodomycosis and actinomycosis.

Protozoal Infections

Toxoplasmosis is important as a cause of encephalitis *in utero* and in the newborn. There is inflammation of the meninges and brain substance, resulting in hydrocephalus and cerebral calcification. The disease in the mother escapes detection although antibodies may be demonstrated in the maternal serum.

Cerebral malaria due to *P. falciparum* (p. 63) and trypanosomiasis (p. 64) are also examples of cerebral protozoal infections.

Worm Infestations

Cysticercosis, the larval form of *T. solium* and hydatid cysts may involve the brain. *Toxocara canis* produces granulomatous inflammation in the brain and in the retina. In trichinosis, the parasite may block small arterioles, causing an acute inflammatory reaction with many eosinophils.

Disseminated (Multiple) Sclerosis

This is a relatively common disease of obscure aetiology that usually develops in early adult life but may present for the first time at any age. It is characterized by a remitting and relapsing course which is gradually progressive. Patchy demyelination occurs particularly in the white matter, the recent lesions appearing pink and the old lesions grey. In the more severe lesions there is loss of axons as well as loss of myelin sheaths. The damaged area is eventually replaced by a glial scar. Cerebellar ataxia, sensory loss, optic atrophy and eventually mental impairment are common manifestations of the disease.

Various aetiological agents have been implicated but none proven. Of recent interest is the similarity of two other demyelinating conditions, kuru and scrapie. Kuru, which causes neurone degeneration as well as demyelination, was discovered in New Guinea in 1952 where it was found to be associated with cannibalism. It is more common in women and children of certain isolated tribes in whom it was the custom to eat human remains. It is believed that some patients dying of kuru were eaten and in this way the disease was transmitted. The disease is now becoming extinct due to the abolition of cannibalism. Scrapie is a demyelinating disease of sheep. A similar disease is found in old mice. Both kuru and scrapie are believed to be transmitted by an infective agent and this raises the possibility of similar infective agents for other demyelinating diseases including multiple sclerosis.

Subacute Combined Degeneration of Cord

This is a serious complication of pernicious anaemia and is the reason why treatment of the disease with vitamin B_{12} must be persistent and adequate.

Demyelination of the posterior and lateral columns of the cord result without subsequent gliosis. The most common symptoms of the disease are paraesthesiae in the hands and feet with loss of vibration sense. Later there may be spasticity of the limbs with manifestation of upper motor neurone disease.

Other Nutritional Deficiencies

These include Wernicke's encephalopathy due to thiamine deficiency, and pellagra due to nicotinic acid deficiency. Wernicke's encephalopathy occurs in chronic alcoholics. The lesions are found in the mammillary bodies, the walls of the third ventricle, aqueduct and fourth ventricle. They consist of brown discoloration and haemorrhages associated with endothelial proliferation of small vessels. Pellagra causes gastrointestinal, neurological and cutaneous lesions. The latter consist of scaly erythema and pigmentation. In the alimentary tract there is glossitis and inflammation of the oesophagus, stomach and intestine leading to diarrhoea. In the brain there is loss of ganglion cells in the cortex and basal ganglia of the brain and anterior horn cells of the cord. There is commonly a peripheral neuritis. These deficiencies are often complicated by other vitamin deficiencies.

Parkinson's Disease

This is also known as paralysis agitans. It may be a sequel of encephalitis lethargica but more commonly it is of unknown aetiology, developing in elderly people. There is tremor and limb rigidity. Histologically there is vacuolation and destruction of nerve cells in the substantia nigra and globus pallidus. Surgical destruction of the globus pallidus or the dorsolateral portion of the thalamus abolishes the tremor.

Syringomyelia

This disease is of uncertain aetiology. The cord is most commonly enlarged in the cervical region by a cyst containing yellow fluid and surrounded by glial scar tissue. The cyst does not communicate with the spinal canal and is not lined by ependyma. Pressure on the sensory and later the motor pathways leads to loss of sensation especially for heat and pain, and upper motor neurone signs in the legs. Charcot's joint may develop in the shoulder.

Tumours

These are classified as shown on page 117. Primary tumours of the brain are less common than secondary tumours, the most important metastatic tumours in the brain being from carcinoma of the lung and breast. Metastatic deposits of carcinoma are most commonly situated in the cerebral hemisphere at the junction of the grey and white matter. They are usually multiple, well defined and reproduce the histological features of the primary tumour. Haemorrhage into the necrotic centre of the tumour is a common terminal event. Cerebellar metastases are about half as common as those in the cerebral hemispheres. Metastatic tumour in the meninges may result in seedling deposits throughout the subarachnoid space. The CSF will have a raised cell count and tumour cells may be identified.

Glioma

Astrocytoma accounts for most gliomas. It arises anywhere in the brain or spinal cord but is found most frequently in the cerebral hemispheres in adults and in the cerebellum in children. The tumour may become cystic and this is seen most often in the childhood cerebellar tumours. Haemorrhage and necrosis are common in the more malignant varieties. Astrocytomas may be graded according to their degree of differentiation, but this varies in different parts of the tumour and grading may be misleading in small diagnostic biopsies. The best differentiated are ill-defined tumours that may produce increased firmness of the brain and enlargement of one hemisphere. The edge of the tumour may be impossible to identify and histologically there may be great difficulty in distinguishing this from reactive gliosis. These tumours tend to recur after attempted excision and cause death usually within a few years. At the other end of the scale, highly malignant astrocytomas show greatly increased cellularity, pleomorphism, mitoses and vascular proliferation with prominent endothelial cells. These highly malignant tumours used to be called *glioblastoma multiforme*. They may reach massive size and cause death within a few months of diagnosis. Haemorrhage and necrosis are features of these more malignant tumours.

Oligodendroglioma is very much less common than astrocytoma. They occur in adults usually in the frontal lobes and are rare in children. These tumours tend to be well differentiated and slow growing with focal areas of calcification which may facilitate their radiological localization. Less commonly more malignant variants may be impossible to distinguish from other highly malignant gliomas. Histologically these tumours consist of neat, box-like, cells with clear cytoplasm giving a honeycomb appearance.

Ependymoma is a slow-growing tumour that occurs mostly in children and young adults. They arise from the walls of the ventricles or spinal canal, most commonly the fourth ventricle. Most of these tumours consist of epithelioid cells arranged in rosettes. A papillary pattern of growth may be found and this is often accompanied by a myxomatous stroma—myxo-papillary ependymoma. These papillary tumours should be distinguished from benign choroidal papillomas which are common in children and may cause hydrocephalus. Papillomas are difficult to remove and as a result they may recur.

Medulloblastoma is a tumour confined to children. It arises in the midline of the cerebellum from primitive neural tissue before differentiation into neurones and glia. The tumour consists of small dark-staining cells resembling adrenal neuroblastomas and retinoblastomas. Because medulloblastomas are situated near the fourth ventricle there is a risk of obstruction to the flow of CSF resulting in hydrocephalus. These tumours have a very poor prognosis.

Spread of Gliomas

Medulloblastomas show the greatest tendency to metastasize through the subarachnoid space. Other gliomas, even the more highly malignant varieties, do not metastasize outside the central nervous system unless there has been surgical intervention when they may involve the skull and tissues of the neck. They are all locally invasive within the brain and cord.

Vascular Tumours

Vascular malformations (angiomas) in the brain and meninges may be a cause of cerebral haemorrhage. The only true vascular tumour of any importance is the *haemangioblastoma*. This is a cystic cerebellar tumour, found mostly in children. In the wall of the cyst there is usually a nodule consisting of endothelial-lined vascular spaces and lipid-laden foamy cells. These tumours are always well circumscribed and therefore more amenable to surgery than most cerebral tumours. Haemangioblastoma may be associated with retinal angioma and cystic disease of the pancreas and kidney. (Lindau–von Hippel disease).

Meningioma

These tumours arise from arachnoid cells that protrude into dural venous sinuses. The most common sites are along the superior saggital sinus, the sphenoidal ridge, the olfactory groove, the posterior cranial fossa, and along the spinal cord. They are slow-growing, well-defined tumours that compress surrounding structures. Eventually they may invade the overlying bone and stimulate osteoblastic activity causing new bone formation. A variety of histological patterns is described. The common pattern consists of whorls of spindle-shaped fibroblastic cells with concentrically laminated calcified bodies (psammoma bodies). Other meningiomas may appear more vascular. Sarcomatous change is rare.

Meningiomas present mostly in adult life and many are found coincidentally at post-mortem. Because they are attached to the dura and are well-defined, these tumours may be successfully treated by surgery.

Nerve-sheath Tumours

Neurofibroma

These tumours may be single or multiple as in von Recklinghausen's disease. They arise on cranial, spinal and peripheral nerves, causing expansion of the nerve. They are usually ill-defined merging with the surrounding connective tissue. Microscopically, neurofibromas consist of interlacing wavy bundles of delicate fibrils and Schwann cells. Vessels in the tumour are often hyalinized and there may be myxomatous change in the stroma.

Neurilemmoma

These tumours also may be single or multiple and associated with von Recklinghausen's disease (neurofibromatosis). They arise in the same distribution as neurofibromas. Those in the cranial nerves most commonly involve the eighth nerve and are called acoustic neuromas. Spinal tumours may protrude through the vertebral foramina as 'dumb-bell' tumours compressing spinal nerves. On peripheral nerves they may occur in the mediastinum or in the skin. Neurilemmomas are usually well circumscribed. They consist of bundles of fibrils and Schwann cells, the nuclei of which are arranged in rows or palisades. Myxomatous change in the tumour is common. These tumours are less liable to become malignant than neurofibromas.

Neurofibromatosis (von Recklinghausen's Disease)

This is inherited as a Mendelian dominant. It is characterized by multiple neurofibromas and neurilemmomas, *café-au-lait* pigmentation of the skin, optic and cranial gliomas and meningiomas. There is a risk that one or more of these neurofibromas may undergo malignant change.

Neurofibrosarcoma

These tumours behave as fibrosarcomas, infiltrating locally and metastasizing by the blood stream to the lungs. They may arise in preceding neurofibromas or neurilemmomas. Large deep-seated neurofibromas arising on main nerve trunks are more likely to become malignant than superficial tumours. Neurofibrosarcomas most often arise in the leg, posterior abdominal wall or thorax.

Neuroblastoma and ganglioneuroma

These tumours have been previously described (p. 118).

Further Reading

Russell, D. S. and Rubinstein, L. J. (1971) *Pathology of Tumours of the Nervous System*. London, Arnold.

29 The Skin

Inflammatory, allergic, traumatic and other 'medical' diseases of the skin form a specialized field in pathology and will not be considered in this chapter. Certain skin diseases are usually treated by surgical excision of the lesion or may be diagnosed by biopsy. It is these lesions which are seen most frequently in pathology and which the student is more likely to see in histological sections.

Cysts

The term *sebaceous cyst* is often erroneously used synonymously with *epidermoid cyst*. Both appear macroscopically as cysts filled with pultaceous material or hard keratin. Sebaceous cysts are found more commonly on the scalp and anterior chest wall, being derived from pilosebaceous follicles. They are lined by stratified, plump, eosinophilic epithelial cells which do not flatten near the cavity of the cyst. Histologically, the cyst contents consist of amorphous sebaceous material. Epidermoid cysts are lined by stratified squamous epithelium which flattens and keratinizes near the surface, to be shed as keratin into the cyst lumen. Epidermoid cysts may arise by obstruction to the outflow from skin appendages, or they may result from trauma and implantation of epidermal cells into the dermis. Low-grade squamous carcinomas may arise in epidermoid cysts, but they rarely metastasize. Such lesions, may ulcerate to give a fungating mass in the scalp known as *Cock's peculiar tumour*. *Dermoid cysts* are developmental abnormalities and occur at lines of fusion of embryonic clefts. The angle of the eye or mouth are common sites. They resemble epidermoid cysts but also contain pilosebaceous follicles and rarely sweat glands in their wall. *Pilonidal cysts* may occur as a result of obstruction of a pilonidal sinus. This is usually found in the lower part of the back between the buttocks. Ingrowths of epidermis containing hairs may cause irritation following trauma or they may become infected. Frequently, the sinuses are found to track far out from the superficial punctum and wide excision is required to prevent recurrence.

Warts

The common wart, verruca vulgaris, occurs mainly in children but is also seen in adults. They are often multiple, especially on the hands. Those that occur on the feet (plantar warts) become deeply embedded due to the pressure of weight-bearing and may be painful. Condyloma acuminata are warts which occur in the anogenital region and form large, fleshy outgrowths. All these warts are due to virus infection. The common wart consists of hyperplastic squamous epithelium (acanthosis) thrown into papillary folds (papillomatosis) and covered by thickened keratin (hyperkeratosis). Superficial cells in the epidermis become vacuolated and contain keratohyaline granules. Condylomata acuminata do not usually show so much hyperkeratosis and they may have an oedematous connective tissue core infiltrated by plasma cells.

Molluscum contagiosum is another viral infection of the skin resulting in umbilicated nodules a few millimetres in diameter. Histologically they show flask-shaped hyerplasia of squamous epithelium which contains characteristic inclusion bodies within some cells—molluscum bodies. Minor trauma is usually sufficient to cause a host reaction which destroys the lesion.

Keratoacanthoma, also known as molluscum sebaceum, may present as a rapidly growing wart or it may mimic squamous carcinoma. Keratoacanthoma arises on hair-bearing skin as a dome-shaped nodule with a central keratin plug. They may reach a size of two centimetres in the course of a few weeks but usually undergo spontaneous regression in three to six months. In old people, regression is often incomplete and squamous carcinoma may develop. Histologically, keratoacanthoma shows epidermal proliferation with downgrowth of epithelium to form a hemispherical mass. There is surface keratinization to form the keratin plug seen macroscopically. The surrounding epidermis is normal; in this way keratoacanthoma differs from most squamous carcinomas which arise in a field of atypical squamous epithelium, often the result of solar irradiation (solar keratoses).

Seborrhoeic wart is more appropriately called a *basal cell papilloma*. These pigmented papillomas occur most frequently in elderly people anywhere on the skin surface other than the palms and soles. They show basal cell proliferation characteristically raised above the level of the surrounding epidermis. Keratin cysts may form within the basal epithelium. Often there are features of similarity between basal cell papillomas and warty naevi (*naevus verrucosus*) the latter being foci of congenital papillary hyperplasia of the epidermis with overlying hyperkeratosis.

Premalignant Conditions and Carcinoma-in-situ

Irradiation by sunlight is the commonest predisposing factor in producing carcinoma in the skin. X-rays were an important cause in radiologists before the danger was recognized. Tar and certain mineral oils are also important, and there are still many cases of skin cancer due to taking of arsenic in Fowler's solution for skin diseases or as a 'tonic'.

Sunlight produces degeneration of dermal collagen so that it assumes some of the staining characteristics of elastic. The epidermis shows atypical squamous cells and abnormal formation of keratin resulting in *solar keratosis*. This progresses to in-situ carcinoma and eventually to invasive carcinoma.

Leukoplakia occurs as white patches on the oral mucosa, vulva and penis. It results from chronic irritation and histologically shows epithelial proliferation with long downgrowths of epithelium (rete pegs), hyperkeratosis, hyalinization of the superficial dermis and chronic inflammation. Atypia of the surface epithelium progresses to invasive squamous cell carcinoma. This condition should be distinguished from *lichen sclerosus et atrophicus* (p. 238.).

Bowen's disease is a form of intraepidermal squamous cell carcinoma very similar to that produced by arsenic. There is gross atypia of the full thickness of the epidermis, with bizarre giant cells, abnormal mitoses and keratinization of individual cells. The lesions occur as single or multiple red plaques originally described on the trunk but occurring anywhere on the body surface.

Paget's disease of nipple has been described in the chapter on breast diseases (p. 253). Rarely Paget's disease may occur in the anogenital and abdominal skin. Under these circumstances it may be associated with rectal or sebaceous carcinoma.

Basal Cell Carcinoma

This is the commonest malignant tumour in man. It does not metastasize and most are successfully treated so that very few cause death. They may be single or multiple and arise in normal or solar-damaged skin. If untreated basal cell carcinomas infiltrate and eventually erode surrounding structures including bone. Histologically they consist of proliferating basal cells, usually in rounded islands invading the dermis. Less frequently they may become cystic or pseudo-glandular due to mucoid degeneration of dermal collagen. Some are pigmented and may mimic malignant melanoma.

Squamous Cell Carcinoma

Squamous carcinoma very rarely develops in skin which does not show evidence of one of the precancerous lesions already described. They occur mainly on light-exposed areas; those that arise on the trunk are more often associated with arsenical keratoses. They may form a papillary mass or they may ulcerate. The rate of growth varies from case to case as does the degree of differentiation. Usually it is possible on microscopy to see keratinizing 'pearls' of squamous epithelium infiltrating the dermis. In other cases, differentiation may be so poor that the tumour cells are spindle shaped and mimic sarcoma.

Squamous carcinoma differs from basal cell carcinoma in its behaviour for metastatic spread of squamous carcinoma is common to the regional lymph nodes.

Pigmented Naevi and Melanoma

Melanin is produced in the skin by melanocytes which are clear cells found in the basal layer of the epidermis. Melanin is passed from these cells to epithelial cells which, as a result, may appear pigmented. This accounts for the pigmentation seen in some basal cell papillomas and carcinomas. Melanocytes are probably of neuroectodermal origin and migrate from the neural crest to the skin. Some leave the epidermis and come to lie in the dermis as naevus cells. Phagocytic cells are found with melanocytes in these dermal collections and are known as melanophages. The latter can be distinguished from melanocytes by the DOPA reaction. Dihydroxyphenylalanine (DOPA) is used as a substrate to demonstrate the presence of the enzyme tyrosinase which converts DOPA (and tyrosine) to melanin, and this enzyme is found only in the melanin-producing melanocyte.

Pigmented naevi are hamartomatous collections of naevus cells that may be found in the dermis or epidermis. The type commonly found in adults is entirely within the dermis—intradermal cellular naevus. It consists of nests of naevus cells which become gradually sclerosed in the deeper layers. Any pigment within them is confined to the superficial layers. Multinucleate giant cells may also be found in the superficial layers. In children, collections of naevus cells are more commonly found in the epidermis and in the adjacent dermis. These are known as junctional naevi. Mixtures of the two types are called compound naevi. Epidermal proliferation of naevus cells implies immaturity of the lesion and although this is acceptable in childhood and adolescence, it should be regarded with caution in adults. Cellular naevi in the palms and soles remain junctional throughout life. Blue naevi are pigmented fibroblastic lesions which occur deep in the dermis. It is this depth which makes the melanin appear blue. The naevus cells in blue naevi have not migrated to the epidermis and so do not assume the epithelioid features of cellular naevi. Blue naevi rarely become malignant. They are closely allied to Mongolian blue spot found in the lower part of the back in Mongolian races.

Malignant melanoma is a malignant tumour of melanocytes and accounts for half the deaths from malignant tumours of the skin. Some melanomas arise in long-standing cellular naevi, but others show no evidence of a preceding naevus. They may occur anywhere on the body surface, but sites of friction and trauma are particularly important. This is demonstrated in the African Negro; the incidence of malignant melanoma of the soles is much higher in those who remain bare-foot. The primary site may remain small and clinically undetected in spite of massive deposits of metastatic tumour. Most malignant melanomas are pigmented but some are amelanotic. Any recent increase in size of a pigmented skin lesion, especially if accompanied by ulceration and bleeding should always be suspected as malignant melanoma. Histologically, malignant melanoma may show some features of similarity to cellular naevi but they show junctional activity, greater pleomorphism, bizarre tumour giant cells and frequent mitoses. Epidermal invasion carries tumour cells to the most superficial layers of the epidermis. On the deep aspect there is usually a lymphocytic infiltrate in the dermis. This probably represents a host immune reaction to the tumour and is of interest in view of the recent demonstration of serum antibodies to melanoma cells in patients with localized disease. Pigmented cells may be found at all layers and not confined to the surface as in cellular naevi. Lateral extension is very common and an important cause of recurrence following surgical excision. Malignant melanoma always requires excision of a wide zone of apparently normal surrounding skin. Lymphatic spread to regional lymph nodes and blood stream spread to lungs and liver are common.

Not all malignant melanomas grow rapidly and metastasize early. Those that occur on the face in elderly people usually have a fairly good prognosis, but those on the hands and feet are much more sinister. Occasionally proliferation of melanoma cells is confined to the epidermis and is then known as a *malignant lentigo*. This may be regarded as in-situ melanoma. It does not metastasize until it invades the dermis.

Malignant melanoma is very uncommon before puberty. Most rapidly growing melanomas in children undergo spontaneous regression. They are known as *juvenile melanoma*.

Dermal Tumours

Dermatofibroma (histiocytoma, sclerosing haemangioma) is a common dermal 'tumour' that has many features of reactive rather than neoplastic proliferation. It is hard and smooth, producing a rounded swelling in the skin. On cut surface it appears yellow or cream coloured due to the presence of lipid-laden histiocytes. Various names are given to the lesion because at different stages of development vascular proliferation, histiocytic infiltration and fibrosis may be prominent features. They are poorly circumscribed but benign.

Dermatofibrosarcoma protuberans is the malignant counterpart of dermatofibroma. It is a larger lesion and shows greater mitotic activity. There may be infiltration of underlying fat. Recurrence after attempted excision is common but they rarely metastasize.

Leiomyoma may arise in the dermis from arrector pili muscles or from the wall of blood vessels. The latter is more common and gives rise to a rounded tender nodule in the deep dermis and subcutaneous fat.

Neurofibroma and neurilemmoma are both found in the skin. They have been described previously (p. 302).

Glomus tumours are angiomatous malformations which are found in the skin, where they cause small painful nodules. Histologically they consist of vascular channels surrounded by glomus cells. These are small cells with clear cytoplasm probably derived from pericytes. The lesions are richly supplied with nerves which probably accounts for the pain which is the most important clinical feature.

Other vascular malformations found in the dermis include haemangioma and lymphangioma. Rarely angiosarcoma may arise in the skin, and then follows vascular obstruction particularly to lymphatic vessels. Angiosarcomas are highly malignant neoplasms, metastasizing by the blood stream. Multifocal primary angiosarcomas may be found in limbs with chronic lymphoedema. Kaposi's sarcoma presents with multiple skin plaques usually in adults. Histologically the lesions consist of proliferating blood vessels and spindle cells, the nature of which is uncertain. There may be haemosiderin pigmentation due to escape of blood from the small proliferating capillaries. Foci of similar tumours are found in internal organs late in the disease.

Further Reading

Lever, W. F. (1967) *Histopathology of the skin* 4th edn. London, Pitman.

Index